LEAN AND GREEN

COOKBOOK for BEGINNERS

A Guide to Unlocking of Plans 5&1, 4&2&1

with Easy Recipes Ready in Less Than 30 Minutes to Regain

Your Health and Get Back in Shape in Just a Few Weeks!

Laure Leller

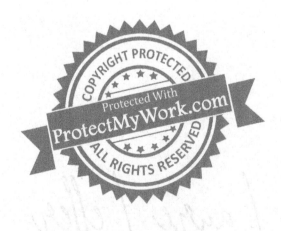

Table of Contents

Introduction..................................6

Chapter 1

Tips For Learning, Knowing, And Succeeding

What exactly is a "Lean and Green diet?...................7

Several weight-loss strategies will be
employed..7

How can a Lean and Healthy Diet help with weight
loss? 8

When it comes to the "Lean and Green" diet, what does
"fueling" mean?...................................9

Benefits of following this diet.................9

Chapter 2

Breakfast Easy Recipes....................10

Chapter 3

Salad and Vegetable Easy Recipes...................26

Chapter 4

Fish & Seafood Easy Recipes...................42

Chapter 5

Poultry Easy Recipes...................54

Chapter 6

Red Meat Easy Recipes...................64

Chapter 7

Dessert Easy Recipes...........................64

Chapter 8

Fueling Hacks Easy Recipes...........................84

Chapter 9

Snacks Easy Recipes...........................98

Chapter 10

Sauces & Dips Easy Recipes.....................110

Chapter 14

PLAN 4&2&1 PROGRAM FOR 28 DAYS......116

PLAN 5&1 PROGRAM FOR 28 DAYS...........118

Conclusion...................................121

INDEX...................................122

This book was written to promote awareness of the importance of paying attention to what one eats and to offer the possibility to vary one's cuisine. However, it is not meant to be a replacement for medical advice. By responding to frequently asked concerns, offering solutions, and offering guidance, it is intended that people can gain a better understanding of eating disorders and what can lead to inadequate nutrition.

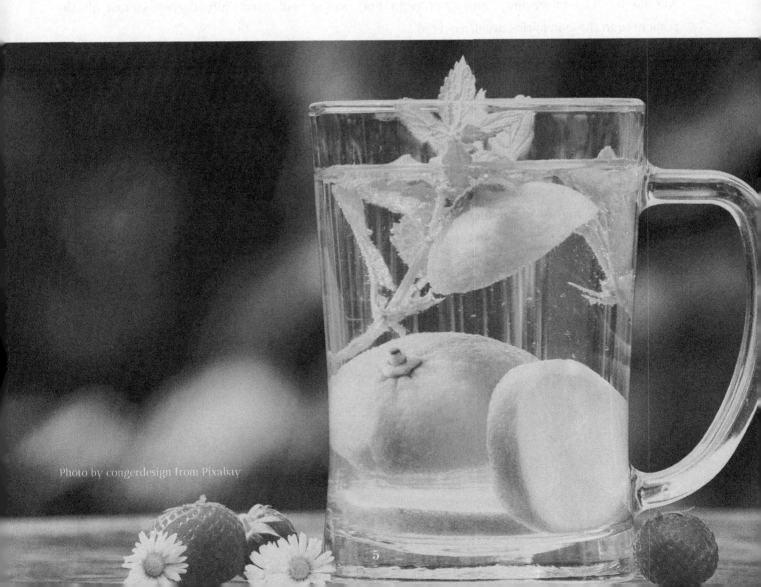

Introduction

Speak with a medical professional about the program before starting a weight loss regimen. In this book, I offer advice solely to help your body and mind function harmoniously. Understanding this will facilitate your ability to observe daily progress. Additionally, it can aid in achieving a healthy weight and identifying the path to lifelong change.

I know she is wary of subjecting her body to daily diet trials while striving to maintain the best possible physical condition. She has stopped eating her favorite foods, started exercising, and has limited herself to bland, boiled items. Yet ultimately, she will experience discouragement. However, now that she has picked up this book, she knows it won't disappoint her. But before embarking on the journey toward a lean, green diet, she must have a fundamental understanding. How will it affect a person's life if they know what they are doing, what they will accomplish, and how they will do it? The uncertainty regarding right and wrong will drastically decrease once all the responses to these inquiries are discovered

This book was created not to restrict or make their healthy lifestyle difficult. Instead, they will experience a sense of organization and positive physiological responses. After starting a diet, people often find that their taste preferences have changed. However, that's not the case with this program.

This book will offer the necessary guidance before beginning a diet because understanding its purpose is essential to completing a task. It will become an enjoyable and exciting endeavor if you are aware of your challenges and the methods required to overcome them.

Properly prepare for the upcoming trip, and you will see that you will never go back
Be sure to never substitute your primary care physician's recommendations for a diet plan.

Chapter 1
TIPS FOR LEARNING, KNOWING, AND SUCCEEDING

What exactly is a "**Lean and Green**" diet?

This meal plan includes ideal amounts of proteins, lipids, and carbohydrates. However, it's necessary to calculate the total. The meal plan should include 150–200 g of lean meat to meet the protein requirement. While it's preferable to obtain protein from meat-free sources like tofu, it's acceptable if that's not possible. A diet plan should be convenient and satisfying, not forced upon you. Additionally, ensure you consume the correct proportions of fiber, vitamins, and minerals daily. Non-starchy vegetables are an excellent way to obtain all three nutrients. Consume these non-starchy vegetables in moderation, aiming for three servings.

Fat is the third essential component that should be part of your meal plan. At this stage, it's important to have a comprehensive understanding of fats and their varieties, something many individuals are unaware of but crucial for dietary concerns. Good and bad fats, also referred to as beneficial and detrimental cholesterol, are two distinct types. Good cholesterol aids in hormone production, does not accumulate in blood vessels, does not contribute to heart-related issues, is vital for organ health, and does not cause heart-related conditions. On the other hand, unhealthy fats should be avoided as they are harmful to the body.

What should I eat, and what shouldn't I eat? After exploring the topic above, you now understand what should be included in your meals. However, it's crucial to know the resources available for obtaining your nutritional requirements. While many resources provide essential nutrients, they may also contain undesirable substances. Therefore, it's important to discern what is relevant and choose the best source to meet your needs.

Several weight-loss strategies will be employed:

Each of the three G&L meal plans advocates eating every two to three hours and consuming approximately two liters of water daily. Vegetable consumption is crucial; experts recommend five servings daily. Limit your daily intake of protein items to 200 grams. Full-body exercises should be incorporated, but it's advisable to consult with your general practitioner before starting.

The 5&1 Plan: this strict diet plan, which must be followed until a healthy body weight is achieved, requires a caloric intake of just 800 to 1,000 calories per day, divided into five meals. Two meals should be spaced apart by a maximum of 2-3 hours. This book provides a range of options for choosing your preferred meals for the day.

The 4&2&1 Plan is ideal due to its flexible eating schedule and its role in helping her achieve a healthy weight. All food groups, including fruits, dairy, carbohydrates, smoothies, bars, pancakes, etc., can be included. It is recommended to consume 4 healthy meals throughout the day, including two lean and green dinners, and one healthy snack, with a 2-3 hour gap between each meal.

The 3&3 Plan is another effective option that involves eating three fuel meals and three L&G (lean and green) meals daily, separated by two to three hours. You can maintain a balanced diet with options such as chicken, desserts, and other foods.

Keep in mind to adhere to these fundamental rules for success:

1. Eat every two to three hours.

2. Consume 1.5 to two liters of water each day.

3. To reduce the stress of dieting, ensure you get eight hours of sleep each night.

4. Perform workout sessions targeting all muscle groups for at least 30 minutes per day, especially at home.

5. Consume 200 grams of protein-rich foods daily, such as Greek yogurt, low-fat cheese, meat, fish, and eggs.

6. Eat five servings of fruits and vegetables each day.

How can a Lean and Healthy Diet help with weight loss?

A "Lean and Green" diet is a well-researched strategy developed through extensive research. The results have been excellent, which is why once someone decides to follow this diet, they find it difficult to stop.

This diet plan requires a total daily calorie intake of 800-1000 calories. With that in mind, you must maintain either the 5&1 plan or the 4, 2&1 plan. When you provide your body with a low-calorie and low-carbohydrate diet, it will start burning the stored fat in your body, leading to weight loss. However, there are some important considerations in this case.

Firstly, you cannot follow this diet for an extended period as it can deplete all your fat reserves, which could be detrimental to your health.

To maintain balance, you should take vacations every six weeks and indulge in fatty foods for three to four days before resuming your routine. These days are often referred to as cheat days.

When it comes to the "Lean and Green" diet, what does "fueling" mean?

"Fueling" refers to obtaining essential carbohydrates, proteins, and calories from a natural, clean diet to meet your body's daily requirements"

To fulfill your body's needs while following a lean and healthy diet, you should consume 3–4 fuelings daily such as cereals, smoothies, cakes, pastries, etc.

Benefits of following this diet

- It is both flavorful and nutritious at the same time.

- You could maintain your diet at a great price.

- There are no needless limits or situations that would ruin your mood.

- Your body will continue to purify, and your stomach and bowels will be content and proper.

- Refueling will retain your energy all day.

- Most importantly, you may take advantage of all these benefits of eating naturally occurring foods.

BREAKFAST
Easy recipes

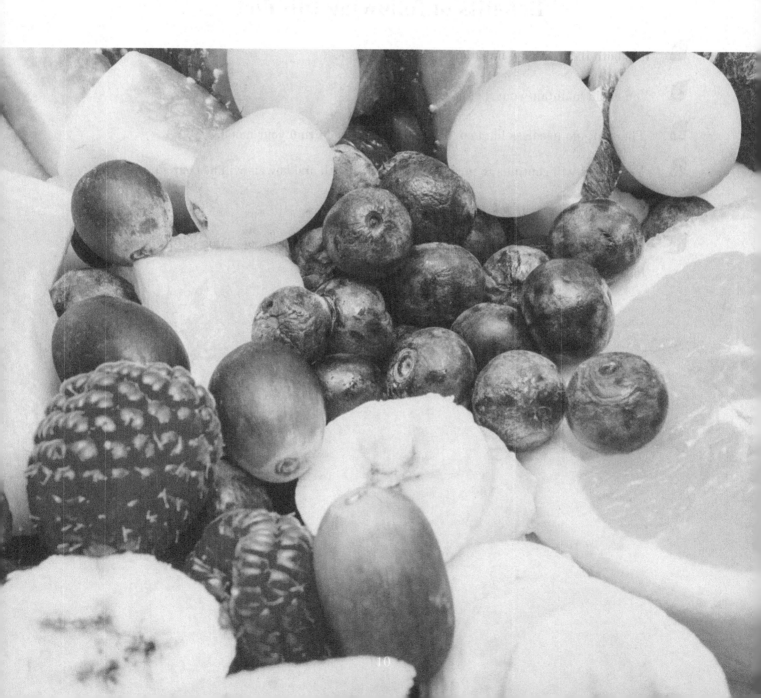

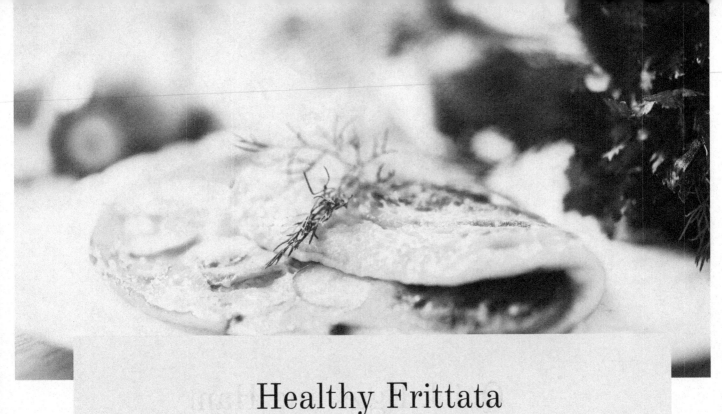

Healthy Frittata

L&G count: 1 green, 2 condiments

SERVINGS: 2   PREPPING TIME: 2 MINS   COOKING TIME: 8 MINS

Ingredients

Six eggs

4 tbsp of unsweetened almond milk

1 tsp of Stacey Hawkins Roasted Garlic Oil

½ cup of sliced green zucchini

½ cup of sliced Portobello mushrooms

1 tbsp of Stacey Hawkins Garlic & Spring Onion Seasoning

Salt to taste

NUTRITION FACTS PER SERVES

Calories 155 kcal

Total Fat 7 gm

Total carbohydrates 3 gm

Protein 17 gm

Directions

1. Add the eggs with almond milk to a bowl, then add a pinch of salt.
2. Heat an 18-inch skillet on the stove.
3. Over moderate heat, pour the roasted garlic oil and add zucchini and mushrooms.
4. Add a bit of salt.
5. Add the egg mixture and proceed to cook for 3 minutes
6. Please turn off the burner and cover it with a lid and leave for 5 minutes

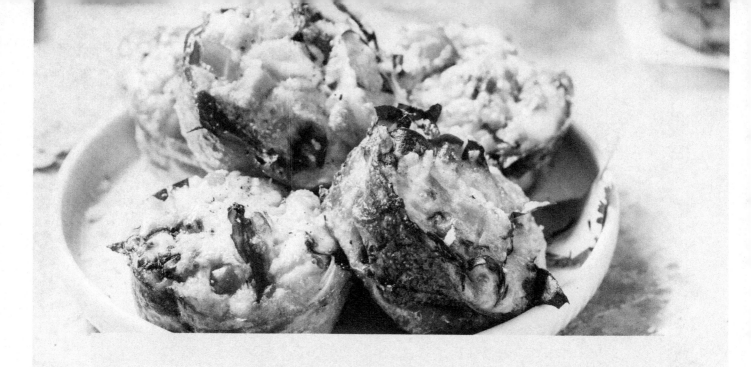

Quick Eggs and Ham

L&G count: 2 greens, 1 condiment, 2 healthy fats

SERVINGS: 2   PREPPING TIME: 15 MINS   COOKING TIME: 30 MINS

Ingredients

two tbsps butter
one large leek finely
shredded.
1 red bell bell pepper,
finely shredded

1 cup thick-cut ham, sliced
finely into 2-3 cm pieces
a huge handful of arugulas
4 eggs
4-5 tablespoons aged
cheddar, grated.

NUTRITION FACTS PER SERVES
Calories 164 kcal
Total Fat 2 gm
Total carbohydrates 9 gm
Protein 8 gm

Directions

1. In a saucepan, heat the butter until bubbles appear.
2. When they appear, stir continuously while cooking the bell pepper and leek for three minutes.
3. Add the arugula and ham and continue stirring till the mixture thickens.
4. Include the eggs in the vegetables and mix well.
5. Fill the spaces with the mix in a muffin pan, then sprinkle cheddar cheese.
6. Heat for a total of fifteen minutes at 375°F in the oven.
7. Serve and enjoy

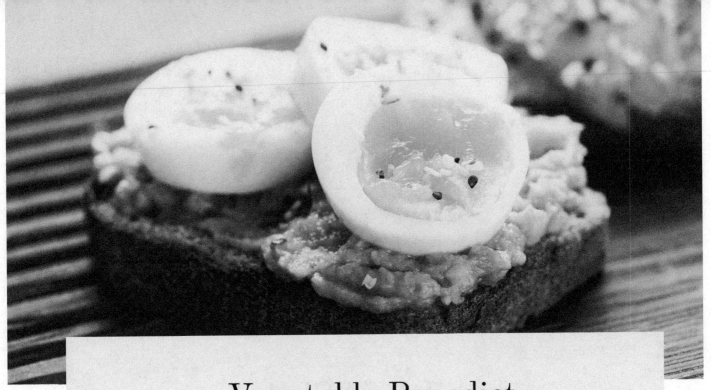

Vegetable Benedict

L&G count: 1 green, 1 condiment

SERVINGS: 3   PREPPING TIME: 8 MINS   COOKING TIME: 8 MINS

Ingredients

3 ripe avocados

Olive oil

½ teaspoon poppy seeds

4 gluten-free black
bread toast

3 eggs

1 lemon

NUTRITION FACTS PER SERVES

Calories 220 kcal

Total Fat 1 gm

Total carbohydrates 5 gm

Protein 18 gm

Directions

1. Make the sauce for avocado.
2. Squeeze out the pulp and mash it with a fork in a bowl, adding the lemon juice as well as a dash of salt.
3. Boil eggs in water for 4 minutes.
4. The bread is toasted in a cooking pan.
5. Serve the toasted bread topped well with avocado sauce as well as the eggs

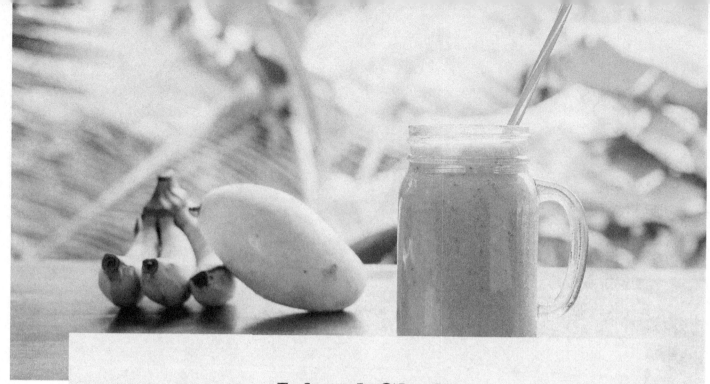

Island Shake

L&G count: 1 green, 1 condiment

SERVINGS: 1   PREPPING TIME: 5 MINS   COOKING TIME: 0 MIN

Ingredients

half a cup of apple cider

2 scoops protein powder

½ cup pineapple

1 mango

1 banana

Ice as per your requirement

NUTRITION FACTS PER SERVES

Calories 122 kcal

Total Fat 2 gm

Total carbohydrates 6 gm

Protein 28 gm

Directions

1. Blend each ingredient thoroughly after adding it to the blender.
2. Ice can be added, but uniformity must be maintained.

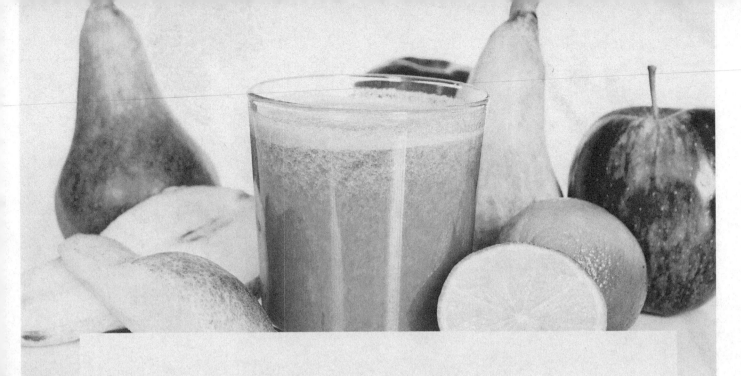

Apple Pear Shake

L&G count: 1 green

SERVINGS: 1   PREPPING TIME: 6 MINS   COOKING TIME: 0 MIN

Ingredients

One cups apple juice   ½ pear
2 scoops protein powder   A few drops of lemon
1 apple   Ice as per your requirements

NUTRITION FACTS PER SERVES

Calories 160 kcal

Total Fat 3 gm

Total carbohydrates 10 gm

Protein 28 gm

Directions

1. Blend each ingredient thoroughly after adding it to the blender.
2. Ice can be added, but be cautious and consistent.

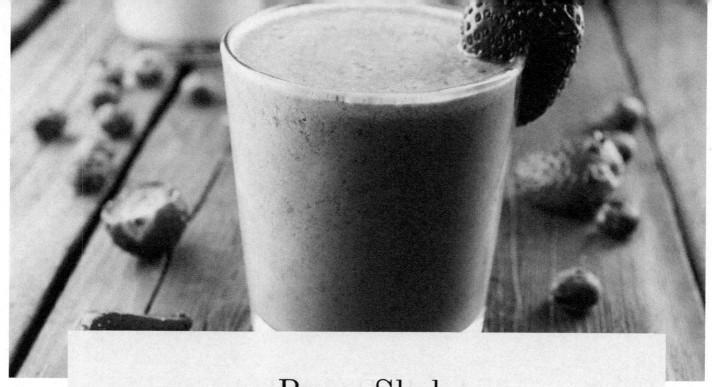

Berry Shake

L&G count: 1 condiment

SERVINGS: 1   PREPPING TIME: 5 MINS   COOKING TIME: 0 MIN

Ingredients

1half a cup of apple cider   4 oz. strawberries

2 scoops protein powder   Ice as per your requirement

½ cup berry

NUTRITION FACTS PER SERVES

Calories 188 kcal

Total Fat 5 gm

Total carbohydrates 19 gm

Protein 20 gm

Directions

1. Blend each ingredient thoroughly after adding it to the blender.
2. Ice can be added, but be cautious and consistent.

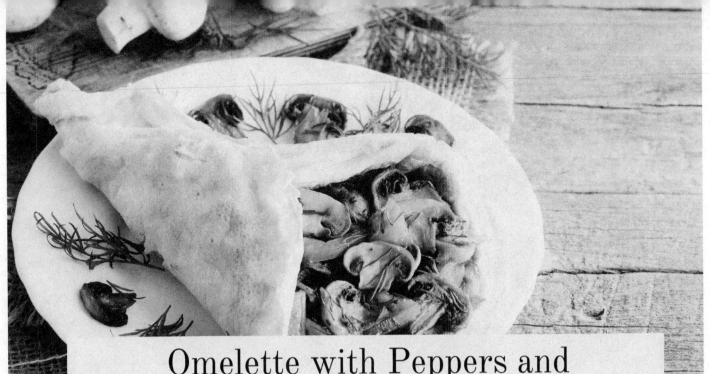

Omelette with Peppers and Mushrooms

L&G count: 1 green, 1 healthy fat, 1 condiment

SERVINGS: 2   PREPPING TIME: 10 MINS   COOKING TIME: 10 MINS

Ingredients

118 fl. oz. olive oil
One-third cup red peppers,
One-third cup onions
Half cup mushrooms

One and a half cups eggs (just the white part)
2 oz. of mozzarella cheese
Garlic, pepper, and dill

NUTRITION FACTS PER SERVES
Calories 165 kcal
Total Fat 19 gm
Total carbohydrates 10 gm
Protein 17 gm

Directions

1. Red peppers, mushrooms, onions, and olive oil should all be cooked together in a skillet until the vegetables are tender.
2. The filling, pepper, and garlic should be added to the pan with the beaten egg white portion.
3. While cooking the egg until the center is no longer firm, place the cheese only on one part and flip it over.
4. Serve.

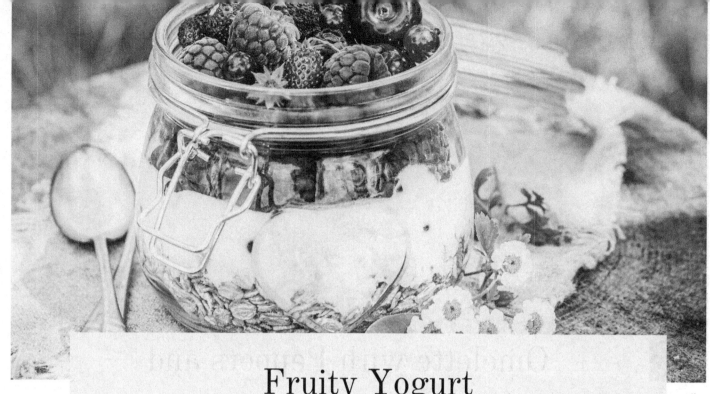

Fruity Yogurt

L&G count: 1 healthy fat, 1 condiment

SERVINGS: 2   PREPPING TIME: 5 MINS   COOKING TIME: 0 MIN

Ingredients

Two cups of raspberries

2 ½ cups oz. blueberries

4 oz. of cherries

2 cups of fat-free yogurt

1 cup gluten-free granola

NUTRITION FACTS PER SERVES

Calories 194 kcal

Total Fat 7 gm

Total carbohydrates 15 gm

Protein 25 gm

Directions

1. In a bowl, layer the yogurt over the fruit.
2. Granola toppings should be garnished.

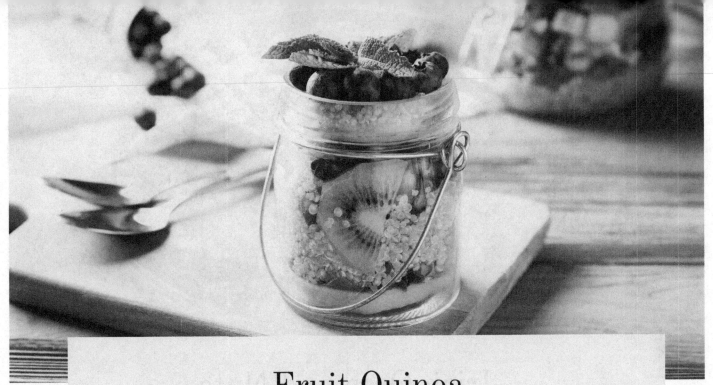

Fruit Quinoa

L&G count: 2 condiments

SERVINGS: 4   PREPPING TIME: 10 MINS   COOKING TIME: 2 MIN

Ingredients

32 ounces of water
2 cups gluten-free quinoa
1 teaspoon cinnamon
¼ teaspoon nutmeg

¼ cup cranberries
¼ cup cranberries
1 kiwi
1/2 peach
Almond milk and honey as needed.

NUTRITION FACTS PER SERVES
Calories 189 kcal
Total Fat 2 gm
Total carbohydrates 7 gm
Protein 30 gm

Directions

1. Quinoa, nutmeg, cranberries, blackberries, sliced kiwi, and chopped peach are added to boiling water in a pot.
2. Cook till the water is all gone.
3. Add the milk as well as honey toppings before serving.

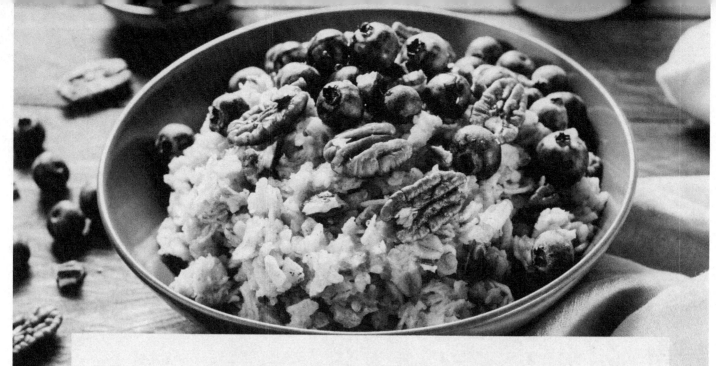

Irish Oats and Nuts

L&G count: 1 condiment, ½ healthy fats

SERVINGS: 2 PREPPING TIME: 5 MINS COOKING TIME: 30 MINS

Ingredients

32 oz. of water

1 cup Irish oats

1/8 cup pecans

1/8 cup of dates and cranberries

One scoop of protein powder

1 teaspoon honey

¼ cup rice, almond milk

NUTRITION FACTS PER SERVES

Calories 197 kcal

Total Fat 2 gm

Total carbohydrates 9 gm

Protein 8 gm

Directions

1. Oats are added to boiling water in a pan and cooked for thirty min.
2. Add your preferred dried fruits, including pecans and apples, and turn the heat off.
3. Add protein powder, then drizzle milk and honey on top before serving.

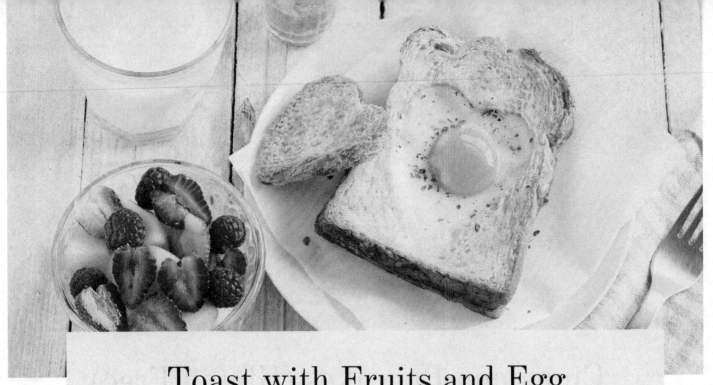

Toast with Fruits and Egg

L&G count: 1 condiment, 1 healthy fat

SERVINGS: 2   PREPPING TIME: 10 MINS   COOKING TIME: 5 MINS

Ingredients

½ teaspoon olive oil

4 eggs

Add salt and pepper to your liking.

Gluten-free bread for toast

2 cups mixed strawberries and apple

NUTRITION FACTS PER SERVES

Calories 224 kcal

Total Fat 2 gm

Total carbohydrates 9 gm

Protein 8 gm

Directions

1. Two eggs should be cracked into the pan, lubricated with olive oil, then scrambled and cooked.
2. Sprinkle a little pepper and salt over the egg after spreading the cheese.
3. Toast the bread, then sprinkle the fruit on it.
4. Serving strawberry garnish

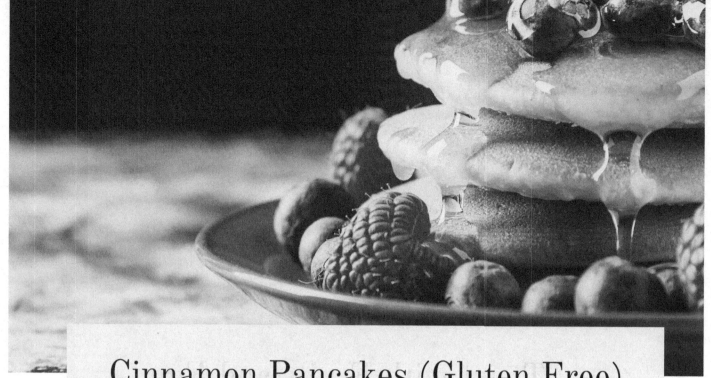

Cinnamon Pancakes (Gluten Free)

L&G count: 2 condiments, 1 healthy fat, 1 leaner

SERVINGS: 2   PREPPING TIME: 10 MINS   COOKING TIME: 5 MINS

Ingredients

One tablespoon organic cream

½ apple

1/2 cup soy flour

½ cup rice flour

1 teaspoon cinnamon

1 cup baking powder

One cup rice or soy milk

1 egg

2 teaspoons honey

1 tablespoon walnut oil

Raspberry and blueberry fruit toppings

Salt

NUTRITION FACTS PER SERVES

Calories 156 kcal

Total Fat 12 gm

Total carbohydrates 10 gm

Protein 34 gm

Directions

1. Apple slices should be heated in an oil-coated pan until tender.

2. Mix the flour, salt, and baking powder in another basin.

3. Put the rice, milk, eggs, honey, and walnut oil in a separate bowl.

4. The two components should then be combined to form a thick batter.

5. Cook the pancake till it is browned after pouring the batter and walnut oil into the pan.

6. Add maple syrup on top.

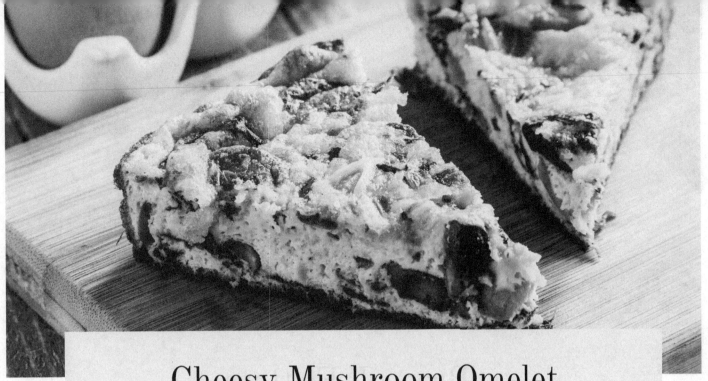

Cheesy Mushroom Omelet

L&G count: 2 condiments, 1 healthy fat, 1 green

SERVINGS: 2   PREPPING TIME: 10 MINS   COOKING TIME: 10 MINS

Ingredients

One tsp olive oil

½ cup mushrooms

½ cup frozen spinach

4 eggs

Salt and pepper

Shredded Cheese

Organic Preserves

NUTRITION FACTS PER SERVES

Calories 224 kcal

Total Fat 2 gm

Total carbohydrates 9 gm

Protein 8 gm

Directions

1. Oil should be heated in a pan at a medium temperature. Add the mushrooms and spinach. For three to four minutes, cook.

2. Cook with moderate heat for 4 minutes after beating eggs with salt and pepper

3. Put cheese on it

4. Serve with bread after folding one side over the other.

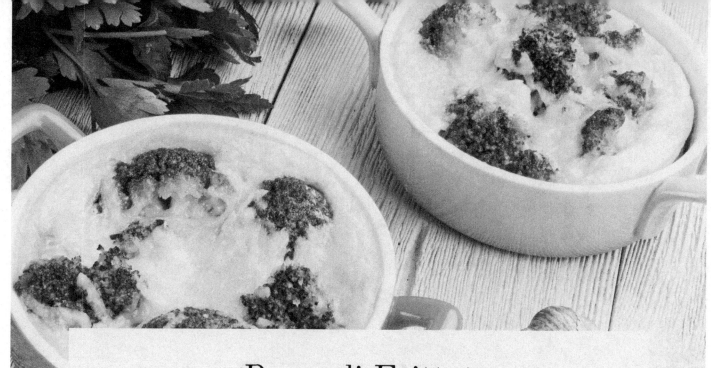

Broccoli Frittata

L&G count: 1 healthy fat, 1 green

SERVINGS: 2   PREPPING TIME: 10 MIN   COOKING TIME: 25 MIN

Ingredients

Two tsps olive oil

2 cups broccoli

Eight eggs

Salt and pepper to taste

½ cup organic cheese

NUTRITION FACTS PER SERVES

Calories 150 kcal

Total Fat 6 gm

Total carbohydrates 6 gm

Protein 19 gm

Directions

1. The oven must be set preheated.
2. Include the broccoli and cook for ten minutes after rubbing the pan with olive oil.
3. In baked ceramic containers, grease them and place eggs adding salt and pepper.
4. Add the cooked broccoli and cheese.
5. Put the dish in the oven and bake it for fifteen minutes at 356 °F.
6. Serve and enjoy

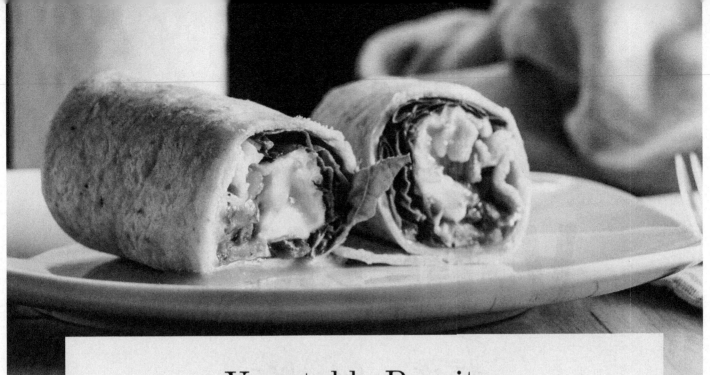

Vegetable Burritos

L&G count: 1 healthy fat, 3 condiments

SERVINGS: 2   PREPPING TIME: 10 MINS   COOKING TIME: 10 MINS

Ingredients

One and 20 fl. ounces olive oil

4 ounces of lettuce

Four eggs

2 tomatoes

Salt & pepper

Four tbsps. cheese

4 corn tortillas

1 jalapeno

NUTRITION FACTS PER SERVES

Calories 97 kcal

Total Fat 13 gm

Total carbohydrates 10 gm

Protein 19 gm

Directions

1. Sauté the tomatoes and jalapeno for five minutes.
2. Whisk the eggs and include them in the tomatoes to create a combination. You can use salt and pepper to taste to season.
3. Each corn tortilla should be heated in the oven for twenty seconds before adding the lettuce leaf and egg mixture to finish with the cheese
4. Roll up the tortillas and enjoy

SALADS & VEGETABLE
Easy recipes

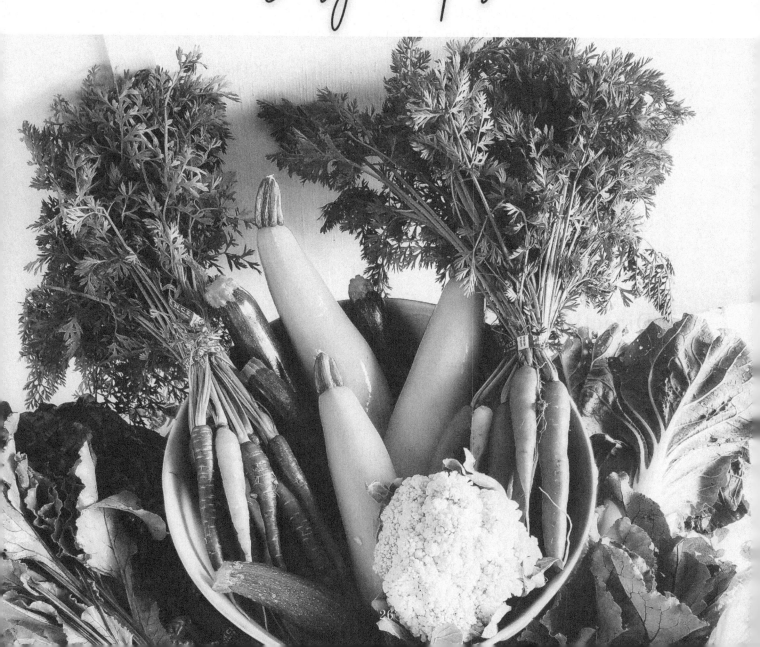

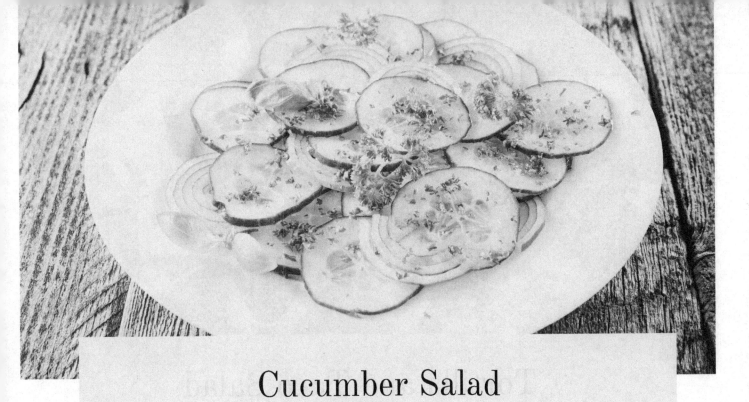

Cucumber Salad

L&G count: 1 green, 1 condiment

SERVINGS: 4   PREPPING TIME: 15 MINS   COOKING TIME: 0 MIN

Ingredients

Four cucumbers peel

One and a half red
onions

1 tbsp Hawkins seasoning

Two tbsps of apple cider
vinegar

NUTRITION FACTS PER SERVES

Calories 52 kcal

Total Fat 0 gm

Total carbohydrates 11 gm

Protein 0 gm

Directions

1. Bring all components simultaneously inside a container
2. Put the entire components together. Then enjoy.

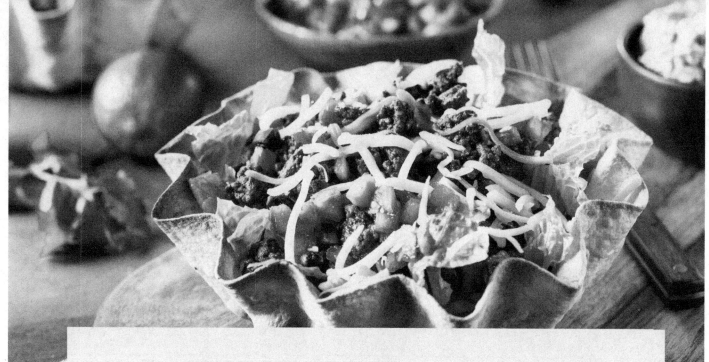

Tortilla and Taco Salad

L&G count: 2 green, 2 condiments, 1 leanest

SERVINGS: 1   PREPPING TIME: 7 MINS   COOKING TIME: 10 MINS

Ingredients

Four oz. ground beef

½ tbsp taco seasoning

3 tbsp romaine tomatoes.

1 shredded romaine lettuce

One tortilla

½ juice of a lemon

1 tbsp grated cheese

NUTRITION FACTS PER SERVES

Calories 103 kcal

Total Fat 7 gm

Total carbohydrates 4 gm

Protein 30 gm

Directions

1. The ground beef should be browned in a pan.
2. Cook for three minutes after adding taco seasoning.
3. Place aside and let it cool.
4. Tomatoes, lettuce, and ground beef should all be combined in a bowl.
5. Fry the tortilla a little, put it inside an empty cup to give it a bucket shape, and grip it tightly with both hands to prevent it from cooling off.
6. Place the prepared topping inside and cover with cheese.
7. Then, toast them a little in the pan and serve.

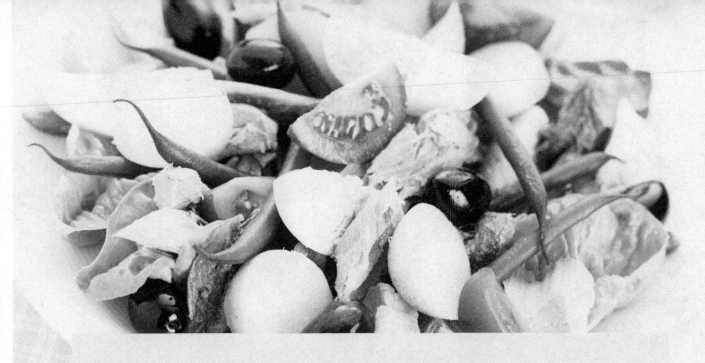

Nicoise Salad

L&G count: 2 green, 2 condiments, ½ leanest

SERVINGS: 1   PREPPING TIME: 12 MINS   COOKING TIME: 0 MIN

Ingredients

Two garlic cloves

2 cans of tuna

2 hard-boiled eggs

3 pitted black olives

2 tbsp of olive oil

3 tbsp of balmy vinegar

½ cup tomatoes

4 cups of mixed greens

1 sliced red onion

1 cup of steamed beans

2 steamed potatoes

NUTRITION FACTS PER SERVES

Calories 96 kcal

Total Fat 7 gm

Total carbohydrates 14 gm

Protein 23 gm

Directions

1. Mix Garlic, oil, and vinegar in a bowl.

2. Then sprinkle the prepared mixture over the tomatoes, mixed greens, beans, boiled eggs, red onions, olives, and tuna in a separate bowl.

3. Now, toss the potatoes in the bowl. After dicing them then, serve

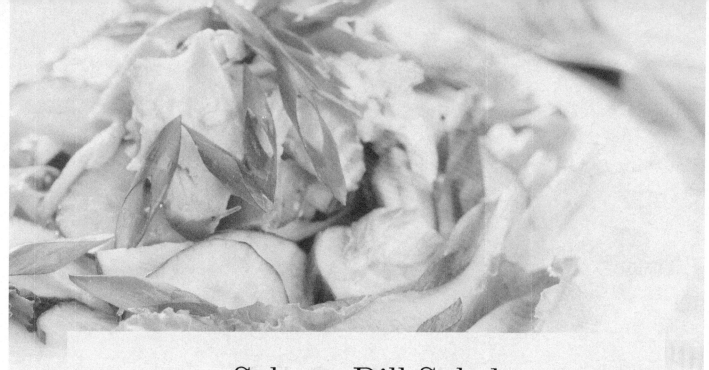

Salmon Dill Salad

L&G count: 2 green, 2 condiments, ½ lean

SERVINGS: 3   PREPPING TIME: 5 MIN   COOKING TIME: 10 MIN

Ingredients

10 oz. cucumbers.

Apple cider vinegar, 4 tablespoons

black pepper, ground, 1/2 tsp.

12 teaspoon of salt

8 oz. salmon fillet

1 tsp zaatar

1 lemon

4 lettuce leaves

NUTRITION FACTS PER SERVES

Calories 108 kcal

Total Fat 8 gm

Total carbohydrates 8 gm

Protein 4 gm

Directions

1. The oven temperature must be set at 300°F
2. The first four ingredients should be combined in a mixing dish.
3. Set a baking sheet covered in foil and add fish, then season with zaatar on both sides of the fish.
4. Put it inside the oven and let it bake for ten minutes.
5. Place the mixed salad ingredients over the lettuce leaves.
6. After the salmon is baked, add it with sliced lemon over the salad.
7. Serve and enjoy.

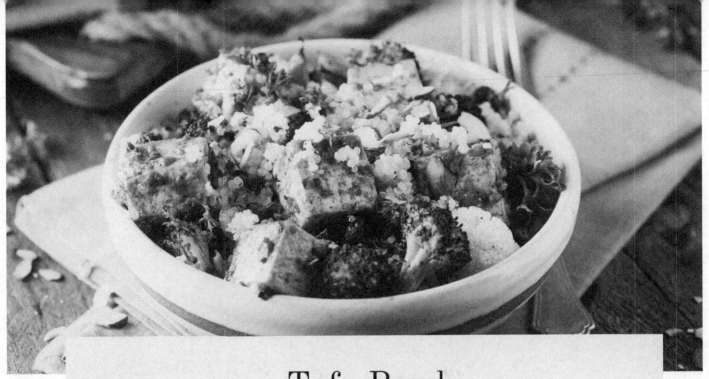

Tofu Bowl

L&G count: 3 green, 2 condiments

SERVINGS: 1   PREPPING TIME: 10 MINS   COOKING TIME: 30 MINS

Ingredients

16 oz. tofu

1 tbsp sesame oil

2 tbsp soy sauce

1 tbsp rice vinegar

¼ cup of quinoa

¼ cup of cauliflower

¼ cup broccoli

¼ cup raisins

NUTRITION FACTS PER SERVES

Calories 80 kcal

Total Fat 16 gm

Total carbohydrates 6 gm

Protein 4 gm

Directions

1. Cover the tofu with a paper towel for 15 minutes, then cut it into cubes.

2. Now sauté the tofu in a pan on shallow heat.

3. After Twelve minutes, eliminate it from the pot and leave it away.

4. For five minutes, sauté the broccoli and quinoa with soy sauce and rice vinegar.

5. Shredded cauliflower and water should be combined in a small bowl and microwaved for three to four minutes.

6. Add the cooked broccoli, cauliflower, and tofu in a serving bowl.

7. Garnish raisins on top and serve.

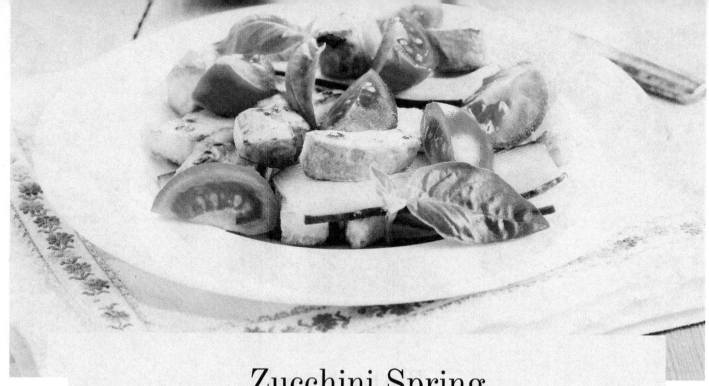

Zucchini Spring

L&G count: 1 green, 2 condiments

SERVINGS: 2   PREPPING TIME: 5 MINS   COOKING TIME: 10 MINS

Ingredients

One and 20 fl. oz.
vegetable oil

Half onion

3 sliced medium
zucchini

Half cup tomatoes

One tbsp any seasoning

Basil for garnish

NUTRITION FACTS PER SERVES

Calories 45 kcal

Total Fat 2 gm

Total carbohydrates 6 gm

Protein 1 gm

Directions

1. On medium flame, onions should be cooked for five minutes until soft and transparent.
2. Before combining the tomatoes and zucchini, seasoning should be added.
3. Cook them for five minutes after tossing them in the pan.
4. Salt and pepper or other seasonings can be added to taste while cooking.
5. After removing it from the pan, garnish it with basil before serving.

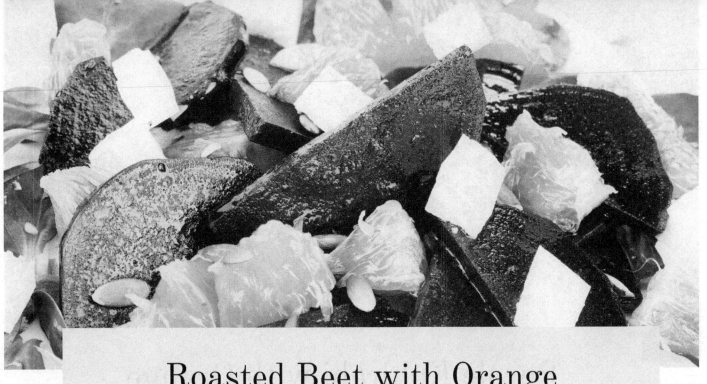

Roasted Beet with Orange

L&G count: 1 ½ green, 1 condiment, 2 healthy fat

SERVINGS: 2   PREPPING TIME: 12 MINS   COOKING TIME: 90 MINS

Ingredients

2 ½ orange

3 red beets

1 cup chopped feta cheese

Olive oil

Salt & pepper

One tablespoon sunflower seeds

NUTRITION FACTS PER SERVES

Calories 109kcal

Total Fat 6 gm

Total carbohydrates 12 gm

Protein 4 gm

Directions

1. Set the oven to 356 °F
2. Cut the stalks after washing the beets in fresh water.
3. Beets should be placed in the oven, covered, and drizzled with olive oil.
4. Roast the beets for one hour until a toothpick can easily pierce them.
5. Remove the peel by gently pressing the sides of the beets with a paper towel.
6. The beets should be cut into one-inch pieces. Cut the oranges into slices
7. Add beets, oranges, diced feta, and a few drops of oil, salt, and pepper as required into a container.
8. Add the toasted sunflower seeds and, as a garnish, valerian salad leaves serve.

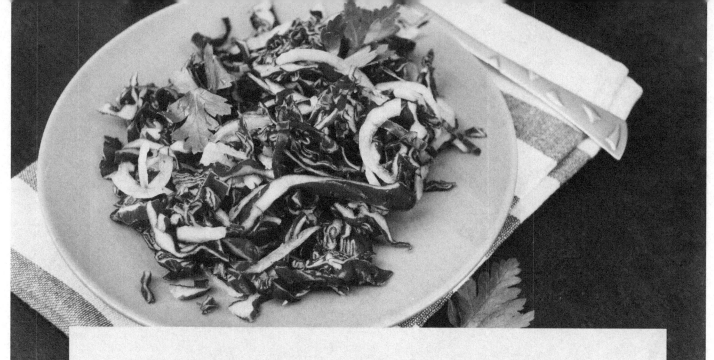

Purple Kohlrabi with Orange

L&G count: 1 green, 2 condiments

SERVINGS: 2   PREPPING TIME: 10 MINS   COOKING TIME: 0 MIN

Ingredients

Two cups shredded
purple kohlrabi

2 tbsp presley

1 tsp of sunrise seasoning

1 tbsp of orange juice

1 tsp of Cajun seasoning

1 lemon juice

1 lime zest

1 orange zest

NUTRITION FACTS PER SERVES

Calories 38 kcal

Total Fat 2 gm

Total carbohydrates 4 gm

Protein 1 gm

Directions

1. Put all the components inside a container except cilantro and kohlrabi.
2. Combine thoroughly and add the shredded kohlrabi.
3. Add a little cilantro and serve.

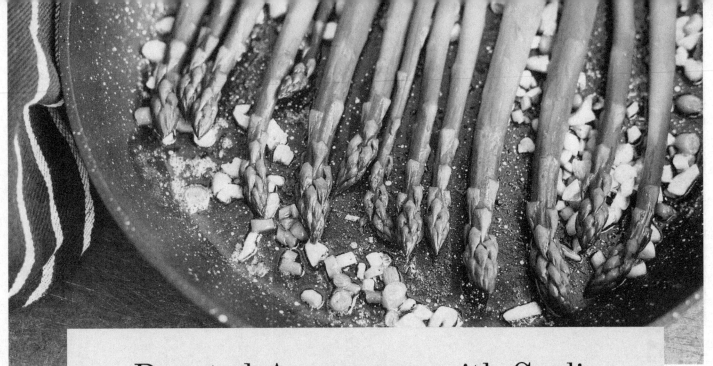

Roasted Asparagus with Garlic

L&G count: 1 green, 2 condiments

SERVINGS: 5   PREPPING TIME: 3 MINS   COOKING TIME: 15 MINS

Ingredients

11 tbsps of oil   16 oz. asparagus
10 cloves of garlic   1 tbsp onion seasoning

NUTRITION FACTS PER SERVES

Calories 48 kcal

Total Fat 2 gm

Total carbohydrates 5 gm

Protein 2 gm

Directions

1. Heat the oil on a high flame inside a pan until it sizzles.
2. Now put garlic in the sizzling oil after mincing it.
3. Then add in the asparagus and seasoning.
4. Cook everything from ten to fifteen minutes.
5. Dish out and serve.

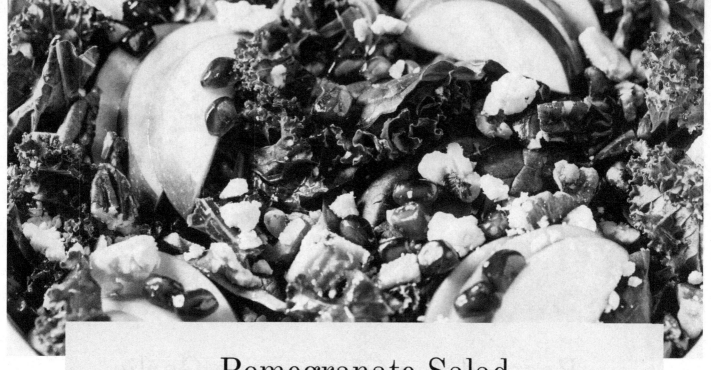

Pomegranate Salad

L&G count: 1 condiment

SERVINGS: 4   PREPPING TIME: 16 MINS   COOKING TIME: 0 MIN

Ingredients

One tbsp balsamic
vinegar

1 tbsp avocado oil

A dash Hawkins
seasoning

1 tsp Dijon mustard

2 tbsp. grated goat cheese

8 oz. of green salad

2 red apples

2 tbsp. walnuts

4 tbsp pomegranate seeds

NUTRITION FACTS PER SERVES

Calories 90 kcal

Total Fat 4 gm

Total carbohydrates 8 gm

Protein 3 gm

Directions

1. Add the first five ingredients to a bowl.
2. These should be whisked together until smooth.
3. Add the greens, apples, and walnuts in a serving bowl, then combine them with the dressing.
4. Garnish with some pomegranate seeds and serve.

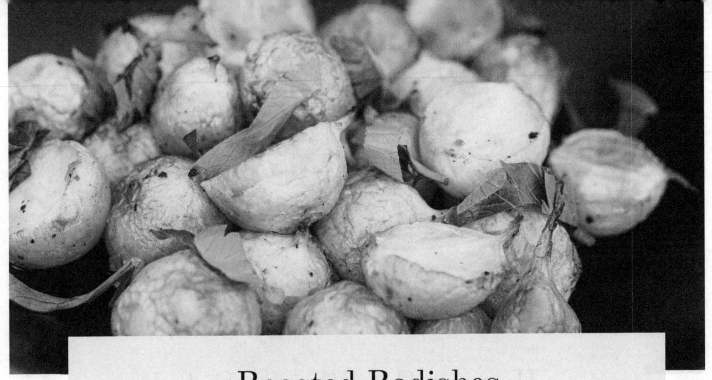

Roasted Radishes

L&G count: 2 condiments

SERVINGS: 4   PREPPING TIME: 5 MINS   COOKING TIME: 30 MINS

Ingredients

16 ounces of radishes

2 tablespoon of oil

1 tsp of dill seasoning

1 tsp of lemon juice

Parsley

NUTRITION FACTS PER SERVES

Calories 39 kcal

Total Fat 2 gm

Total carbohydrates 3 gm

Protein 8 gm

Directions

1. Set the oven to 356 °F
2. The components should be combined in a bowl except for the radishes
3. Coat the radish with the mix and put them in a roasting pan.
4. Now, bake it for 30 minutes.
5. Serve right away after taking it out of the oven.

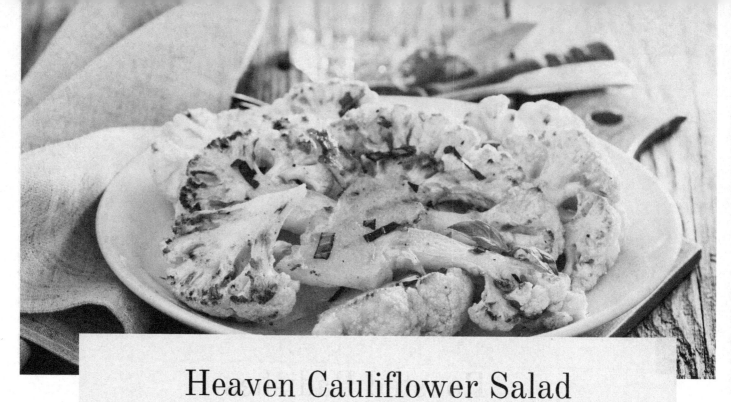

Heaven Cauliflower Salad

L&G count: 1 condiment, 1 green

SERVINGS: 4   PREPPING TIME: 12 MINS   COOKING TIME: 0 MIN

Ingredients

Two cups cauliflower
florets

4 tablespoon of oil

Salt to taste

a pinch of pepper

8 large basil leaves

5 tbsp apple cider vinegar

NUTRITION FACTS PER SERVES

Calories 30 kcal

Total Fat 3 gm

Total carbohydrates 13 gm

Protein 11 gm

Directions

1. Inside a bowl, put all ingredients.
2. Let it sit for thirty minutes.
3. Then serve.

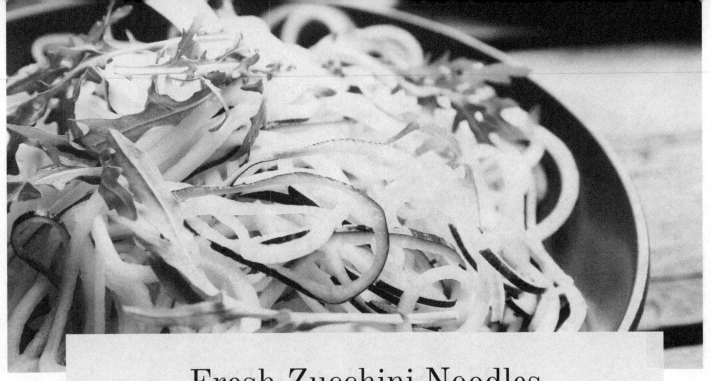

Fresh Zucchini Noodles

L&G count: 1 condiment, 1 healthy fat

SERVINGS: 2   PREPPING TIME: 25 MINS   COOKING TIME: 5 MINS

Ingredients

One tbsp of lemon oil
One and a half cups of
zucchini noodles

1 tbsp Mediterranean
seasoning
1 tsp of Sea salt
Some fresh arugula

NUTRITION FACTS PER SERVES
Calories 115 kcal
Total Fat 1 gm
Total carbohydrates 13 gm
Protein 3 gm

Directions

1. Start with making the zucchini noodles and boil them.
2. Keep them aside when they are boiled.
3. In a cooking pan, add lemon oil over moderate heat.
4. Put noodles and sauté them for a minute when it simmers.
5. Salt and seasonings should be sprinkled; sauté for at least two more minutes.
6. Top it up with fresh arugula.
7. Enjoy after serving.

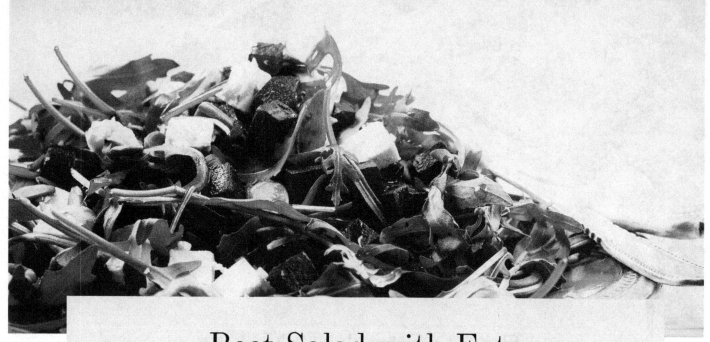

Beet Salad with Feta

L&G count: 1 condiment, 1 healthy fat

SERVINGS: 2   PREPPING TIME: 12 MINS   COOKING TIME: 45 MINS

Ingredients

2 cups of arugula

One steamed beet

Four tbsps. sunflower seeds

Half cup feta cheese.

Olive oil

Salt to taste

NUTRITION FACTS PER SERVES

Calories 37 kcal

Total Fat 2 gm

Total carbohydrates 4 gm

Protein 0 gm

Directions

1. The beet is first diced and then steamed.
2. Take the arugula and chop it.
3. Combine the arugula with the beet, salt, sunflower seeds, and feta in a bowl and season
4. Then serve.

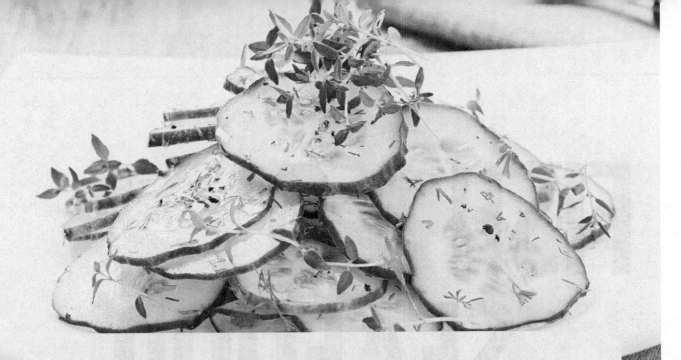

Healthy Quick Cucumber Salad

L&G count: 1 condiment, 1 green

SERVINGS: 3   PREPPING TIME: 10 MINS   COOKING TIME: 0 MIN

Ingredients

Three sliced fresh
cucumbers

1 tablespoon of rice
vinegar

1 teaspoon of sugar

½ tsp of salt

2 tablespoon of chopped
chives

NUTRITION FACTS PER SERVES

Calories 19kcal

Total Fat 0 gm

Total carbohydrates 5 gm

Protein 1 gm

Directions

1. Include sugar, vinegar, salt, sugar, and chives in a bowl and stir well
2. Add sliced cucumbers
3. Serve and enjoy

FISH & SEAFOOD
Easy recipes

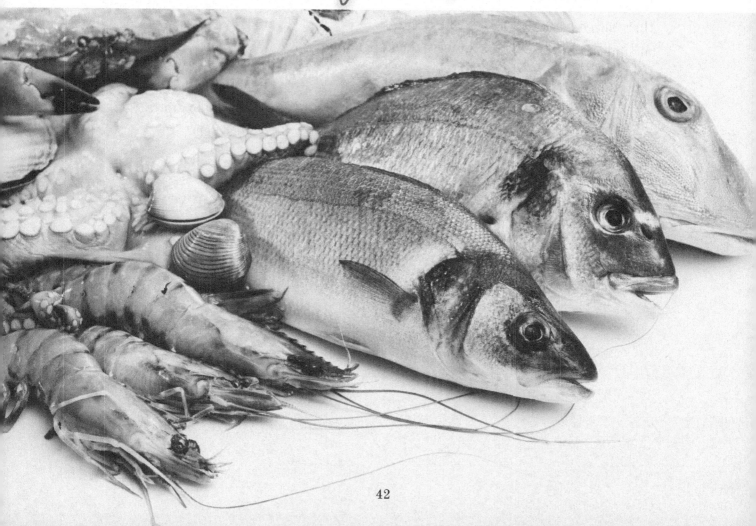

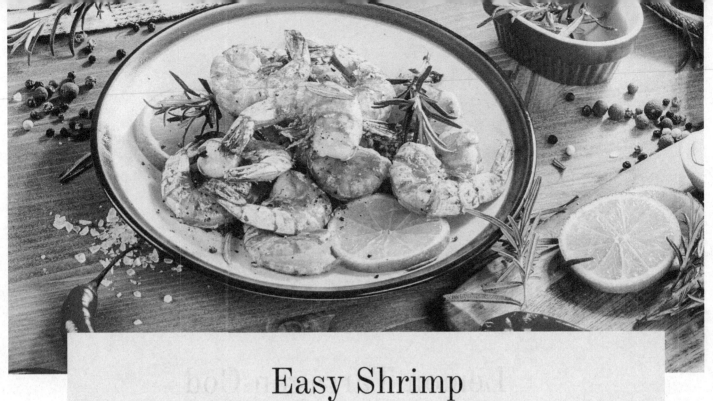

Easy Shrimp

L&G count: ½ lean, 2 condiments, 1 healthy fat

SERVINGS: 4   PREPPING TIME: 13 MINS   COOKING TIME: 17 MINS

Ingredients

½ tbsp onion powder

3 tbsp butter

½ tbsp garlic

½ tbsp salt

2 cups shrimp

One lemon juice

Rosemary

Salt

Black pepper

NUTRITION FACTS PER SERVES

Calories 80 kcal

Total Fat 0 gm

Total carbohydrates 11 gm

Protein 19 gm

Directions

1. In a pan, melt the butter, then add garlic. Now sauté it for one minute.
2. Now add the onion powder, black pepper, lemon juice, and shrimp.
3. 15 minutes should be allowed for cooking, then add the rosemary with salt.
4. Dish out and serve.

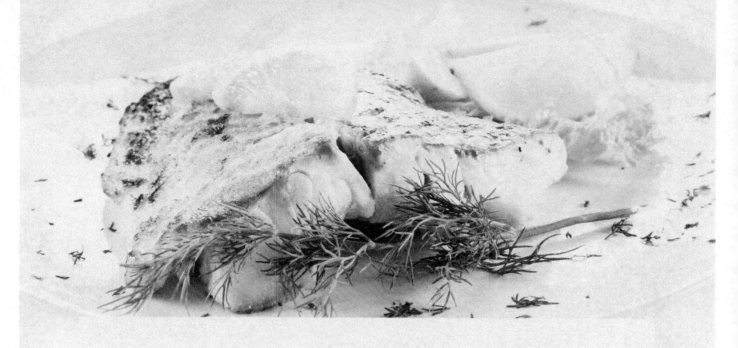

Lemon Tarragon Cod

L&G count: 2 condiments

SERVINGS: 4   PREPPING TIME: 5 MINS   COOKING TIME: 15 MINS

Ingredients

Two and a half cups cod fillets

One tablespoon of lemon oil

One tbsp of ranch seasoning

Red and black pepper

NUTRITION FACTS PER SERVES

Calories 180 kcal

Total Fat 1 gm

Total carbohydrates 0 gm

Protein 43 gm

Directions

1. Heat oil in a pan over moderate flame.
2. Add fish to heated oil.
3. Now put all the seasoning, then sauté each side until browned.
4. Serve and enjoy.

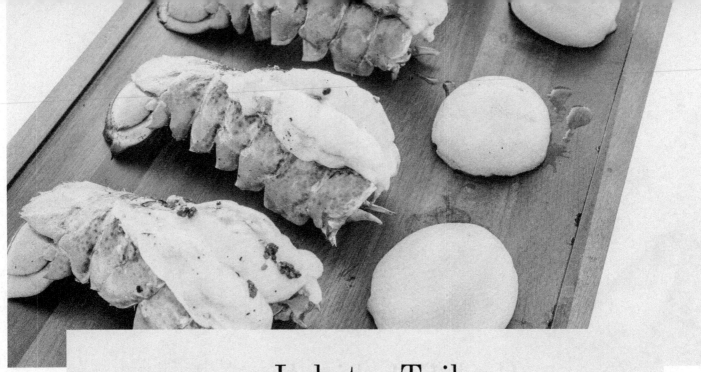

Lobster Tail

L&G count: 1 condiment, 1 healthy fat

SERVINGS: 4   PREPPING TIME: 10 MINS   COOKING TIME: 15 MINS

Ingredients

5 cups lobster tails

Two cups of butter

Lemon wedges

NUTRITION FACTS PER SERVES

Calories 64 kcal

Total Fat 1 gm

Total carbohydrates 0 gm

Protein 14 gm

Directions

1. The lobsters should be defrosted for the necessary period.
2. Heat the oven to 400°F and slice the lobster's top shell to release the flesh from the shell.
3. Put the meat, meat side up, on top of the shell, and lay it on a baking sheet.
4. Top the lobster with butter.
5. 10–12 minutes are needed to bake.
6. Lemon wedges and melted butter are added, then served.

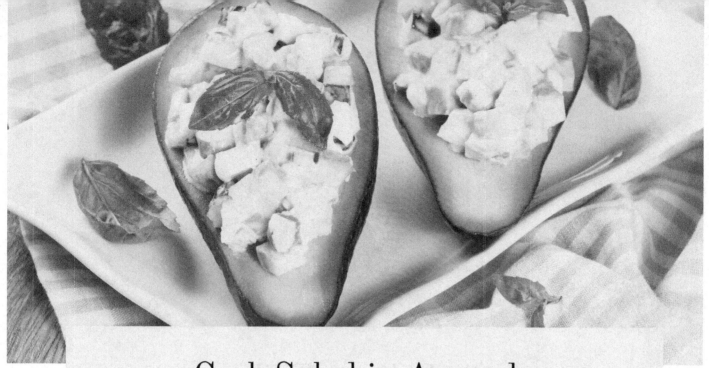

Crab Salad in Avocado

L&G count: 2 condiments, 2 healthy fats, 1 lean, 1 green

SERVINGS: 6   PREPPING TIME: 10 MIN   COOKING TIME: 0 MIN

Ingredients

2 cups of crab meat

Four tbsps of Greek yogurt

2 tbsp of sour cream

1 boiled potato

4 tbsp of celery

Juice of 2 lemons

One tbsp of dill

One tbsp of red onion

One tablespoon of parsley

3 large avocados

1 tsp of sugar

½ tsp of salt

NUTRITION FACTS PER SERVES

Calories 200 kcal

Total Fat 2 gm

Total carbohydrates 38 gm

Protein 13 gm

Directions

1. Chop the celery, onion, and herbs, making a vinaigrette.
2. Cut the avocado halfway, discard the stone, and partially hollow them out before cutting the pulp into cubes. Add lemon juice to the pulp and the remaining avocado cubes.
3. Combine the yogurt, sour cream, salt, sugar, and lemon juice.
4. The crabmeat should be broken up and combined with the vinaigrette, the diced potato, and the diced avocado flesh.
5. The dressing should be placed inside the avocado halves.
6. Keep chilled until ready to serve.

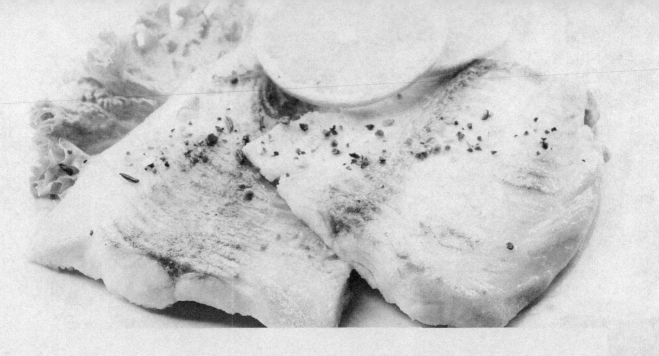

Oven Baked Flounder

L&G count: 1 condiment, 1 green

SERVINGS: 2　　　　PREPPING TIME: 5 MINS　　　　COOKING TIME: 10 MINS

Ingredients

3 flounder filets

One tsp of dill

1 lemon juice

Salt and pepper

½ cup of olive oil

NUTRITION FACTS PER SERVES

Calories 200 kcal

Total Fat 2 gm

Total carbohydrates 38 gm

Protein 13 gm

Directions

1. Include the filets, lemon juice, and seasoning inside a bowl.
2. Mix well.
3. Put the fillets on a prepared baking tray sheet and drizzle the oil over them.
4. Then bake for ten minutes at 392 °F
5. Now serve and enjoy.

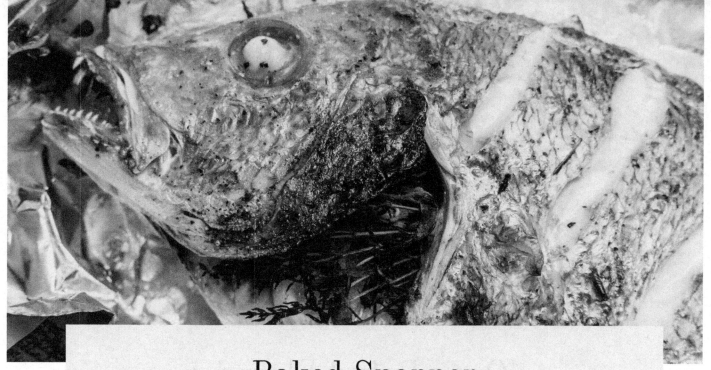

Baked Snapper

L&G count: 1 condiment, 1 healthy fat

SERVINGS: 2   PREPPING TIME: 8 MIN   COOKING TIME: 28 MIN

Ingredients

Two red snappers

½ cup of butter

3 garlic cloves

1 lemon zest

1 lemon

Salt and pepper

NUTRITION FACTS PER SERVES

Calories 109 kcal

Total Fat 1 gm

Total carbohydrates 0 gm

Protein 22 gm

Directions

1. Set the oven to 392 °F
2. Dissolve the butter inside a pan on moderate flame.
3. Cook the garlic in the butter for one minute. Add lemon zest as well.
4. Cut the lemon into slices, then put it in the baking dish.
5. Dry the snapper with a paper towel, then season both sides with salt & pepper.
6. Put the fish over the lemon slices and then top with garlic and butter.
7. Bake it for twenty minutes in the oven.
8. Serve and enjoy.

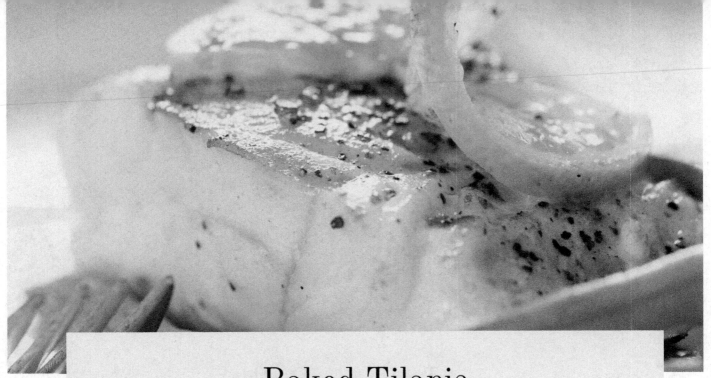

Baked Tilapia

L&G count: 2 condiments

SERVINGS: 2   PREPPING TIME: 10 MINS   COOKING TIME: 15 MINS

Ingredients

4 tilapia fillets

1 tbsp of any seasoning

1 tbsp of olive oil

Half lemon juiced

NUTRITION FACTS PER SERVES

Calories 55 kcal

Total Fat 2 gm

Total carbohydrates 0 gm

Protein 27 gm

Directions

1. Cover the tilapia with oil on both sides.
2. Filets should be placed on a baking tray with seasoning.
3. Oven temperature must be set at 356 °F
4. The fillets should be baked for fifteen minutes.
5. Serve with lemon juice drizzled on top.

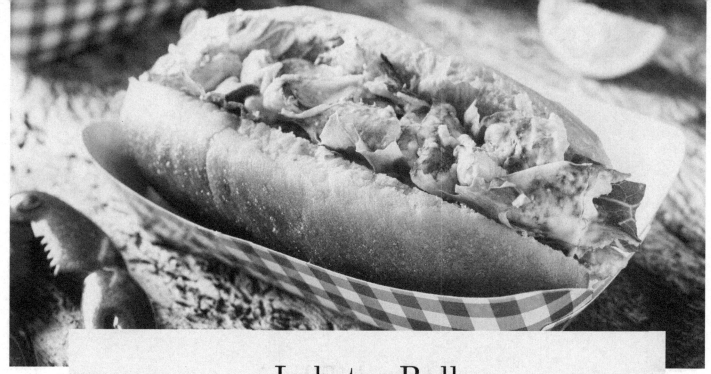

Lobster Roll

L&G count : ½ leaner, 3 condiments, 2 greens

SERVINGS: 2   PREPPING TIME: 20 MINS   COOKING TIME: 0 MINS

Ingredients

One and half cups
cooked lobster meat
¼ cup of cherry
tomatoes
½ celery stalk

4 tbsp of vegan mayonnaise
2 tbsp of green onion
1 tsp of tarragon
½ tsp of lemon juice
½ tsp of black pepper
8 lettuce leaves
4 hot Dog buns.

NUTRITION FACTS PER SERVES
Calories 44 kcal
Total Fat 3 gm
Total carbohydrates 13 gm
Protein 24 gm

Directions

1. Combine the very first eight ingredients in a bowl.
2. Give it a mix
3. Place the leaves on the buns, then top the buns with the mixture.
4. Serve.

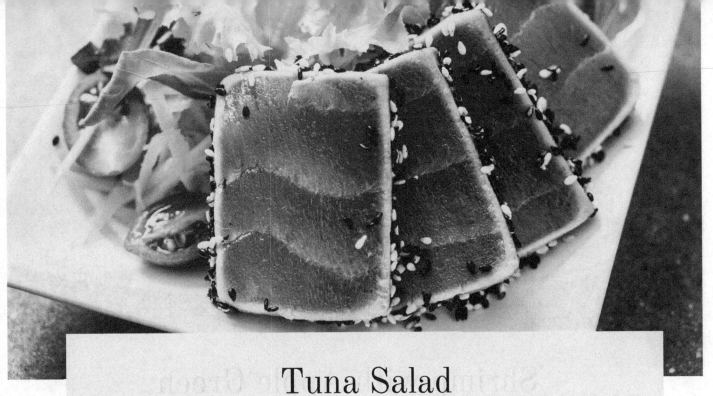

Tuna Salad

L&G count : ½ leaner, 3 condiments, 2 greens

SERVINGS: 3   PREPPING TIME: 5 MINS   COOKING TIME: 0 MINS

Ingredients

3 tuna fillets

4 tbsp poppy seeds

4 tbsp. sesame seeds

1 julienned carrot

1 cup cherry tomatoes

3 tbsp. salsa

4 tbsp lemon juice

½ tsp cayenne pepper

8 oz green salad

Oil and Salt to taste

NUTRITION FACTS PER SERVES

Calories 113 kcal

Total Fat 1 g

Total carbohydrates 19 g

Protein 21 g

Directions

1. Cook the tuna fillets first.
2. Include all the other components in a container and mix thoroughly
3. Now add the tuna on top and serve

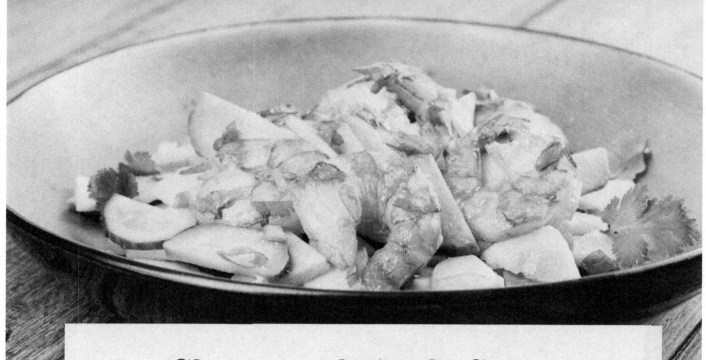

Shrimp with Apple Green

L&G count: 2 condiments, 1 green, ½ lean

SERVINGS: 3   PREPPING TIME: 10 MINS   COOKING TIME: 6 MINS

Ingredients

One tbsp olive oil
Two and a half cups shrimp
2/3 cup avocado
4 tbsp onion

½ cup of parsley
A pinch salt
1½ tbsp lemon juice
2 green apples

NUTRITION FACTS PER SERVES
Calories 90 kcal
Total Fat 2 gm
Total carbohydrates 9 gm
Protein 10 gm

Directions

1. Slice the apples thinly, then set them aside.
2. Combine apples and lemon juice with thinly sliced avocado.
3. Oil should be heated in a pan on moderate flame.
4. Fry the onion in the pan, then add in the shrimp.
5. Sauté the shrimp for Seven minutes.
6. After two to three minutes, turn the shrimp over.
7. Add the shrimp to the apple and avocado mixture, then top with the parsley.

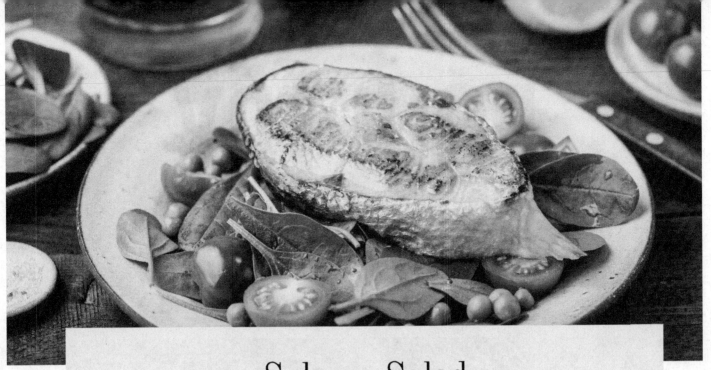

Salmon Salad

L&G count: 1 green, 2 condiments, ½ lean

SERVINGS: 3   PREPPING TIME: 5 MINS   COOKING TIME: 18 MINS

Ingredients

Two cups of baby
spinach
One cup of halved cherry
tomatoes
4 tbsp of apple cider
vinegar

½ tsp of black pepper,
ground
½ tsp of salt
1 cup of skinless, and
boneless salmon fillet
1 tbsp of 3 zaatar
1 medium-sized quartered
lemon

NUTRITION FACTS PER SERVES
Calories 130 kcal
Total Fat 6 gm
Total carbohydrates 4 gm
Protein 26 gm

Directions

1. Warm up your oven to 356 degrees Fahrenheit.
2. Mix the first five ingredients inside a container and toss well to form a salad.
3. Take a baking sheet lined with foil and place salmon onto it. Seasoned from both
sides with zaatar
4. Roast it
5. Serve salad with salmon and lemon

POULTRY
Easy recipes

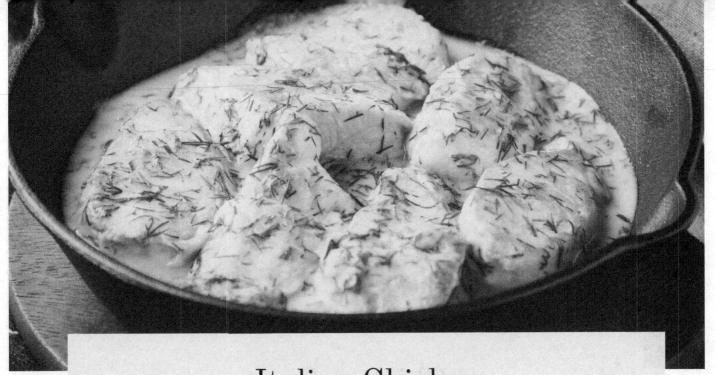

Italian Chicken

L&G count: 1 lean, 3 healthy fats, 1 green

SERVINGS: 3   PREPPING TIME: 15 MINS   COOKING TIME: 28 MINS

Ingredients

35 ounces of chicken
pieces

Two tsps. basil

Two tsps. of oregano

Two tsps. of garlic
powder

3 garlic segment

A handful of herbs

½ cup Greek yogurt

2 lemon wedges

Salt and Pepper

Mozzarella cheese

Parmesan cheese

NUTRITION FACTS PER SERVES

Calories 340 kcal

Total Fat 4 gm

Total carbohydrates 13 gm

Protein 60 gm

Directions

1. First, set the oven to 392 °F.
2. Put cooking spray inside the casserole dish.
3. Put the shredded chicken inside the middle of your casserole dish, and afterward,
top it with oregano and basil.
4. You can season with salt and garlic powder.
5. To the yogurt mixture, add marinara sauce.
6. Spread the yogurt mixture on the chicken.
7. Top with mozzarella and parmesan cheese.
8. For half an hour minutes, bake it.
9. Then serve and enjoy.

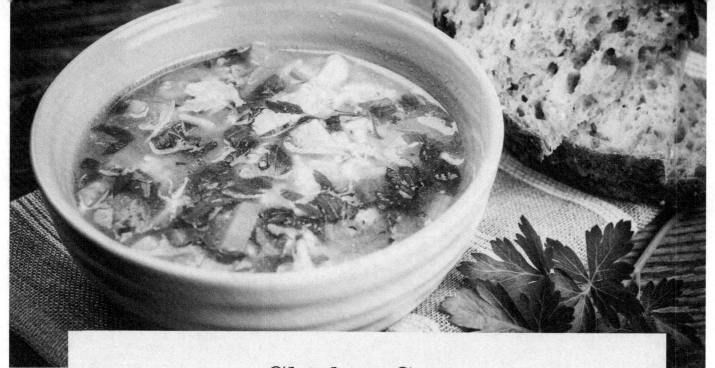

Chicken Soup

L&G count: 2 leans, 3 greens, 2 condiments

SERVINGS: 12   PREPPING TIME: 15 MINS   COOKING TIME: 30 MINS

Ingredients

Two quarters Chicken stock,

20 oz. chicken breast

2 celery stalks

1 cup cut carrots

Quarter cup peas

Half cup green onions

Half cup spinach leaves

One bunch watercress

One cup parsley leaves

One cup basil leaves

1 teaspoon salt

Half teaspoon black pepper

Four to Six cloves of garlic

NUTRITION FACTS PER SERVES

Calories 105 kcal

Total Fat 2 gm

Total carbohydrates 7 gm

Protein 15 gm

Directions

1. Grab a sizable saucepan and fill it with chicken broth.
2. Place the pot on a medium-high burner.
3. Cook the chicken breast for 10 minutes after adding it to the pot.
4. Add the remaining ingredients now.
5. Serve after cooking for about 20 minutes.

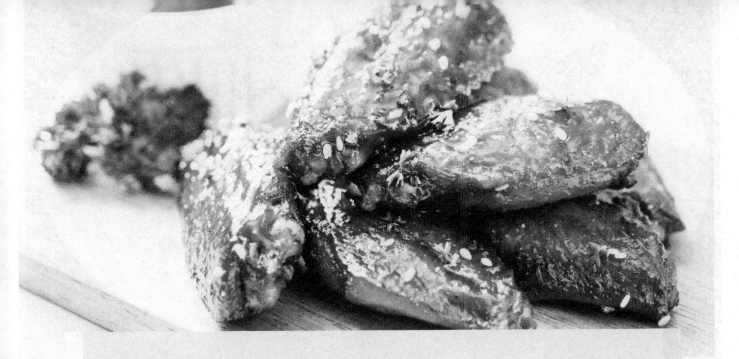

Grilled Chicken Marinated with Beer

L&G count: ½ lean, 1 condiment

SERVINGS: 3   PREPPING TIME: 180 MINS   COOKING TIME: 20 MINS

Ingredients

Can of non-alcoholic beer

2 tablespoons apple cider vinegar

2 tablespoons vegetable oil

70 oz. of chicken wings

2 tbsp. white sesame seeds

Half a cup of soy sauce

NUTRITION FACTS PER SERVES

Calories 170kcal

Total Fat 6 gm

Total carbohydrates 1 gm

Protein 24 gm

Directions

1. Marinate the chicken with the beer, apple cider vinegar, soy sauce, salt, and pepper for at least three hours

2. Warm up the grill.

4. Brush oil on the grill.

5. Grill chicken till it becomes tender.

6. Decorate with white sesame seeds and serve with sauce.

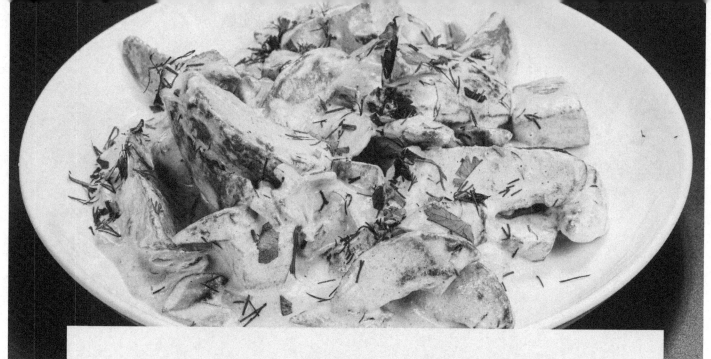

Creamy Chicken Casserole

L&G count: 1 lean, 2 healthy fat, 2 condiments

SERVINGS: 5   PREPPING TIME: 10 MINS   COOKING TIME: 35 MINS

Ingredients

One serving of avocado oil

1 can of chicken soup

70 oz. chicken breast

½ cup greek yogurt

Black pepper

Salt to taste

1/3 cup cheddar cheese

½ cup fresh dill

½ cup fresh parsley

2 cloves of garlic

NUTRITION FACTS PER SERVES

Calories 330 kcal

Total Fat 7 gm

Total carbohydrates 33 gm

Protein 33 gm

Directions

1. Garlic oil is heated in a pan, and garlic is sizzled till it becomes aromatic.
2. Now toss in the dill and sauté them briefly.
3. Mix the broth with the chicken, yogurt, salt, and pepper.
4. Pour this mix into the pan and cook for fifteen minutes.
5. Add cheese, and continue turning while cooking for five minutes.
6. Turn out and serve, decorating with plenty of parsley.

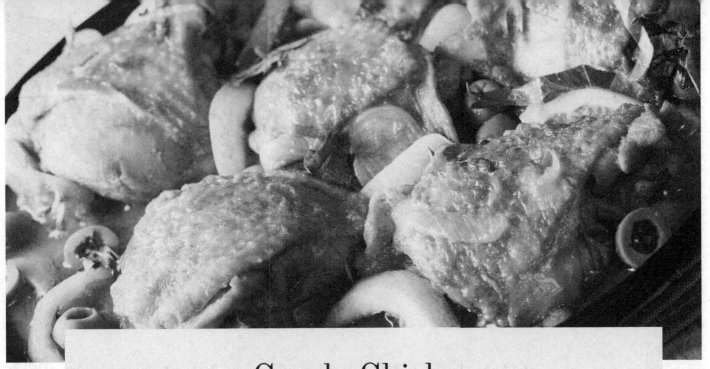

Creole Chicken

L&G count: 1 ½ lean, 1 green, 2 condiments

SERVINGS: 4   PREPPING TIME: 180 MINS   COOKING TIME: 15 MIN

Ingredients

4 chicken breasts

½ cup leeks

2 small cloves of garlic

1.25 cups of chicken broth

1 can of tomatoes

Tomato paste

1 ½ tsp Creole seasoning

¼ tsp cayenne pepper

1 cup green olives

1 ½ cups parsley

1 sliced lemon

NUTRITION FACTS PER SERVES

Calories 380 kcal

Total Fat 12 gm

Total carbohydrates 35 gm

Protein 30 gm

Directions

1. Combine all the ingredients in a crockpot except for the green olives.
2. Cook on a moderate flame for three hours with the lid on.
3. Shred the chicken when it is cooked a little, then leave it on low flame to simmer.
4. Now dish out in a bowl.
5. Add green olives as a garnish before serving.

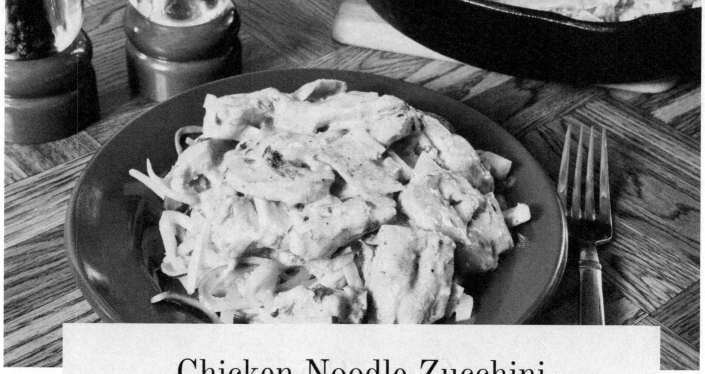

Chicken Noodle Zucchini

L&G count: 1 ½ lean, 1 green, 2 condiments

SERVINGS: 4   PREPPING TIME: 10 MINS   COOKING TIME: 20 MINS

Ingredients

35 ounces of chicken
breast

Two tbsps. of virgin olive
oil

½ cup parmesan cheese

½ tbsp salt

2 oz. vegetable broth

2 medium shallots

2 cups zucchini noodles

2 pinches of parsley

NUTRITION FACTS PER SERVES

Calories 243 kcal

Total Fat 10 gm

Total carbohydrates 6 gm

Protein 30 gm

Directions

1. Shallots should be added to the oil in a pot and cooked for a few minutes until it becomes soft.

2. Add the chicken breast cut and toast it for a few minutes.

3. Add the vegetable stock and parmesan cheese once the sauce has thickened or the chicken is done. Add the fresh parsley to complete.

4. Zucchini noodles are cooked in a pan of salted, boiled water.

5. Put the chicken and noodles in a dish.

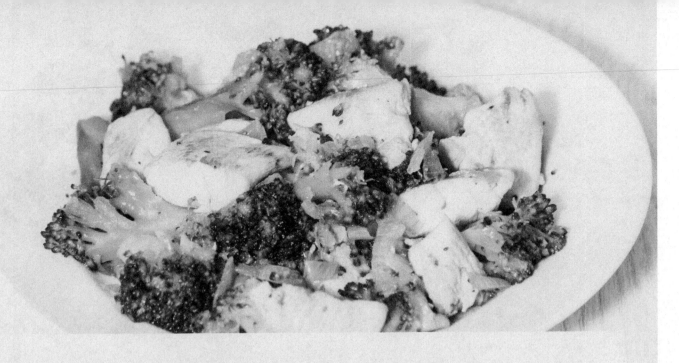

Chicken with Broccoli

L&G count: 1 lean, 1 green, 2 condiments

SERVINGS: 2   PREPPING TIME: 3 MINS   COOKING TIME: 9 MINS

Ingredients

2 tbsp olive oil

One lb. chicken breast

1 cup broccoli

1 tsp sesame seeds

Sliced onions

Soy sauce

Garlic paste

Salt

Pepper

NUTRITION FACTS PER SERVES

Calories 187 kcal

Total Fat 2 gm

Total carbohydrates 21 gm

Protein 35 gm

Directions

1. For three minutes, cook the chicken, cut into pieces, within a pot with one tablespoon of olive oil.

2. Include the broccoli, the rest of the olive oil, and a dash of salt and pepper.

3. After three minutes of cooking, add the garlic paste and soy sauce.

4. Serve topped with sesame seeds and onion slices.

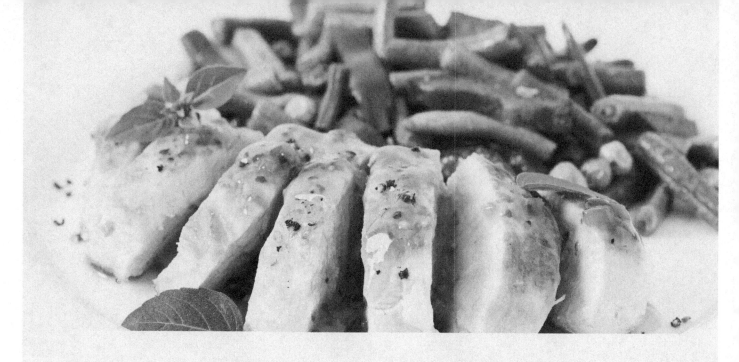

Baked Chicken Breast

L&G count: 1 lean, 1 green, 2 condiments

SERVINGS: 3   PREPPING TIME: 10 MINS   COOKING TIME: 15 MINS

Ingredients

3 boneless chicken
breasts

2 cups green beans

½ cup red bell pepper

One tbsp garlic

One tbsp oregano

Three tbsps olive oil

Salt as required

Pepper as required

Fresh basil

NUTRITION FACTS PER SERVES

Calories 142 kcal

Total Fat 3 gm

Total carbohydrates 0 gm

Protein 27 gm

Directions

1. Set the oven to 350 degrees.
2. Arrange the oil-rubbed dry chicken breast on a sizable baking sheet.
3. Place the already-boiled green beans and bell pepper slices over the chicken breasts.
4. Add oregano and minced garlic to the dish, then add salt and pepper.
5. For twenty minutes, bake.
6. Remove from oven, then leave it for ten minutes.
7. Garnish basil leaves on top and serve.

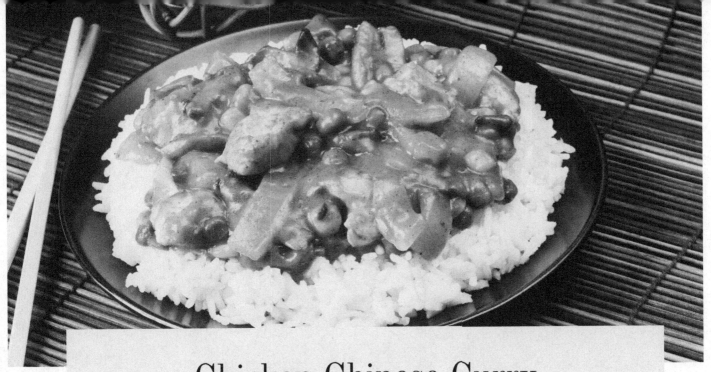

Chicken Chinese Curry

L&G count: 1 ½ lean, 3 condiments, 1 green

SERVINGS: 4   PREPPING TIME: 15 MINS   COOKING TIME: 50 MINS

Ingredients

Skinless chicken pieces

One tbsp corn flour

1 onion

1 garlic

1 tbsp of rapeseed oil

2 cups of boil rice

1 tsp of curry powder

2 pinches of turmeric

One pinch of sugar

1 ½ tsp of ginger

2 cups of chicken stock

Handful frozen peas

1 tsp soya sauce

NUTRITION FACTS PER SERVES

Calories 260 kcal

Total Fat 7 gm

Total carbohydrates 8 gm

Protein 40 gm

Directions

1. Fry onions in a wok with half the oil till soft
2. Include the garlic and cook for a min.
3. Cook for one more minute after adding the sugar and spices.
4. Add soy sauce and chicken stock, then cook for about twenty minutes.
5. Use a hand blender to combine everything.
6. Fry the chicken in the rest of the oil until it turns brown.
7. Add sauce and peas, then cook them.
8. Add water if needed.
9. Serve with the rice when done

RED MEAT
Easy recipes

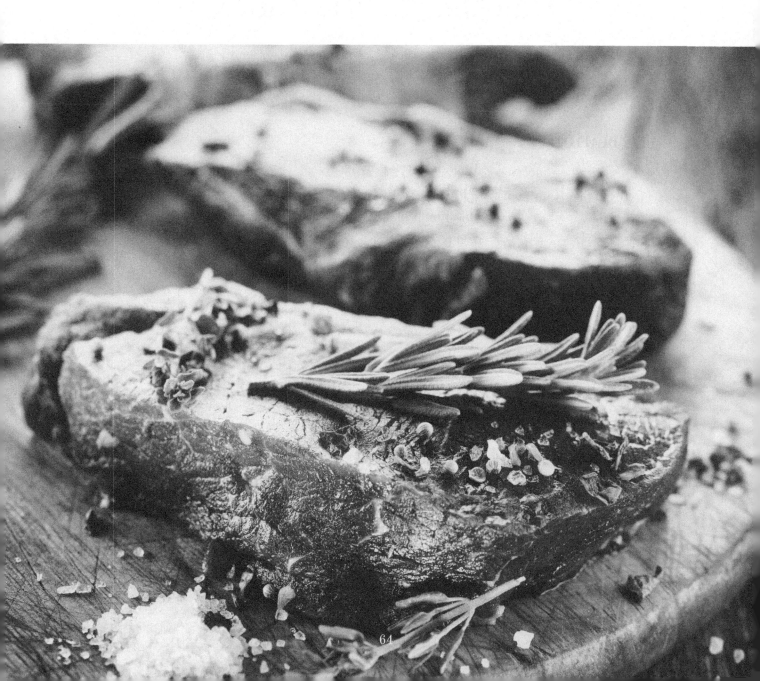

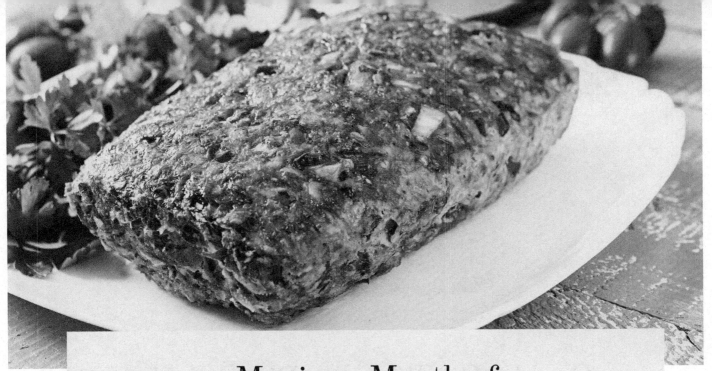

Mexican Meatloaf

L&G count: 1 lean, 3 condiments, 2 healthy fats, 1 green

SERVINGS: 6   PREPPING TIME: 10 MINS   COOKING TIME: 65 MINS

Ingredients

1 cup of beef

Four tbsps of egg powder.

One teaspoon of chili powder

Half teaspoon of cumin

Half teaspoon of salt

2 garlic cloves

¼ cup of salsa

½ cup of Monterey jack cheese

½ cup of cheddar cheese

½ tsp of green chilies

NUTRITION FACTS PER SERVES

Calories 170 kcal

Total Fat 5 gm

Total carbohydrates 9 gm

Protein 21 gm

Directions

1. Set the oven to 370 °F

2. Blend the ground beef with the eggs and seasonings in a bowl. Using wax paper, roll the mixture into a square.

3. Carefully remove the wax paper.

4. Put the loaf in the pan, then add the salsa.

5. For fifty minutes, bake.

6. Place cheese on top and bake once more till it melts.

7. Now serve.

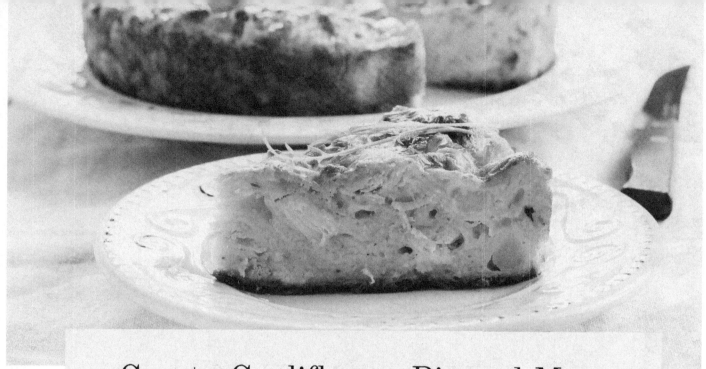

Crusty Cauliflower Pie and Meat

L&G count: 1 lean, 3 green, 3 condiments

SERVINGS: 4   PREPPING TIME: 15 MINS   COOKING TIME: 35 MINS

Ingredients

One and a half pounds of ground beef

One tsp all-purpose seasoning

4 cups vegetables

1/3 cup chicken broth

½ tsp salt and pepper seasoning

2 cups riced cauliflower

4 tbsp cheese

½ tbsp garlic seasoning

Sea salt - olive oil

NUTRITION FACTS PER SERVES

Calories 244 kcal

Total Fat 19 gm

Total carbohydrates 26 gm

Protein 33 gm

Directions

1. Turn the oven on to 370 °F
2. Place a drizzle of oil in a skillet and brown the shredded meat for eight minutes.
3. The vegetables should be cut and cooked for four minutes separately. Add the beef and vegetables after adding the chicken broth and cooking for another five minutes.
4. The cauliflower should be cooked in the microwave for five minutes and crushed
5. Cover the meat and vegetable mixture with the mashed cauliflower, put it in a baking dish, bake for fifteen minutes in the oven, and serve hot.

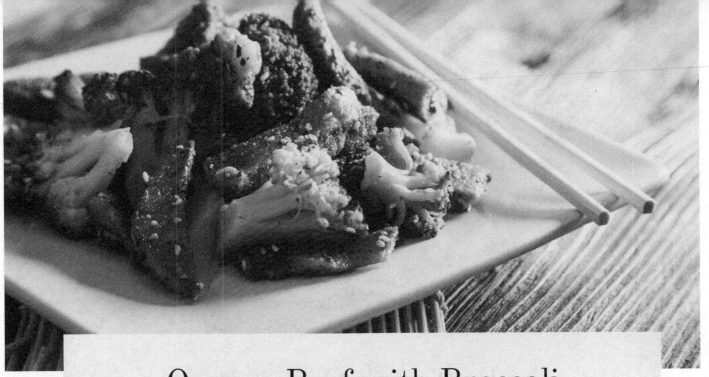

Orange Beef with Broccoli

L&G count: 1 lean, 1 green, 1 condiment

SERVINGS: 4   PREPPING TIME: 10 MINS   COOKING TIME: 10 MINS

Ingredients

One tbsp of orange oil
Two cups of London broil
One capful of wok on
seasoning

Two cups of broccoli
florets
¼ cup of beef stock
Pinch of desperation
seasoning

NUTRITION FACTS PER SERVES

Calories 100 kcal

Total Fat 6 gm

Total carbohydrates 12 gm

Protein 21 gm

Directions

1. In a sizable pan, pour orange oil.
2. sauté meat for three minutes in oil. Add stock, broccoli, and spice. Cover.
3. Cook for five minutes on low flame.
4. Then dish out and serve

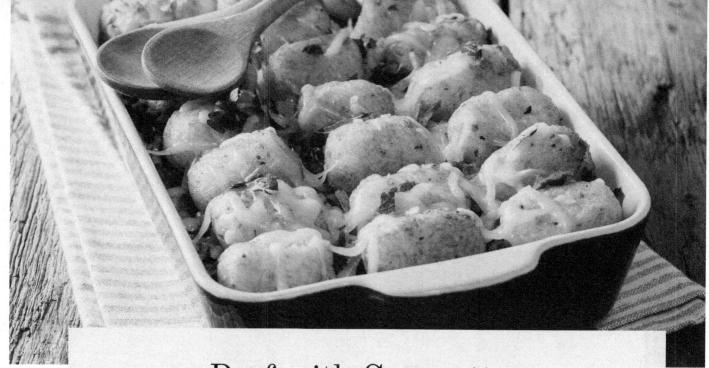

Beef with Croquettes

L&G count: 1 lean, 2 condiments, 2 healthy fats, 2 seasonings, ½ green

SERVINGS: 4   PREPPING TIME: 10 MINS   COOKING TIME: 10 MINS

Ingredients

1-pound beef

One medium onion

½ tsp garlic powder

1 can cream of mushroom soup

1 can cream of chicken soup

One can cream of chicken soup

½ cup milk

½ cup parsley

2-pound bag tater tots

2 cups cheddar Jack cheese

Salt and Pepper as required

NUTRITION FACTS PER SERVES

Calories 157 kcal

Total Fat 1 gm

Total carbohydrates 13 gm

Protein 29gm

Directions

1. Cook the beef until tender and well browned.
2. Combine the garlic powder, soups, milk, and parsley in a mixing dish.
3. Pour this mix into a baking pan.
4. Tater tots should be arranged on the surface of the batter.
5. Seal the baking pot to seal it.
6. Bake for thirty minutes at 250°F until the soup bubbles. After that, please remove it from the oven.
7. Lastly, top the tater tots with cheese and bake again for ten more minutes.
8. After that, garnish with some parsley and serve.

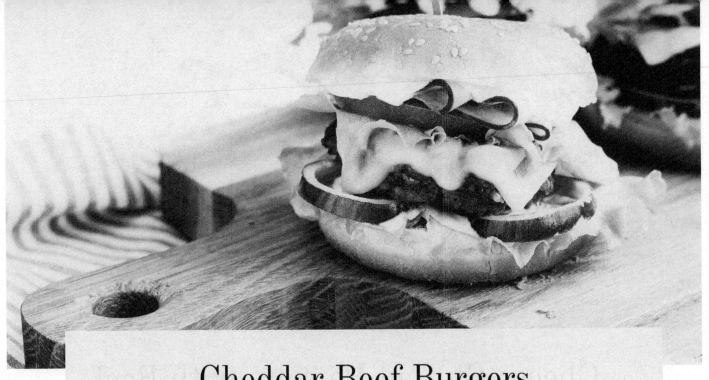

Cheddar Beef Burgers

L&G count: 1 lean, 2 healthy fats, 1 condiment

SERVINGS: 4   PREPPING TIME: 10 MINS   COOKING TIME: 14 MIN

Ingredients

Three cups of lean beef
Half a thinly sliced red onion.
½ tsp of salt
½ tsp of pepper
½ cup of cream cheese
4 tbsp of cheddar cheese

Half tsp of garlic powder
1 diced jalapeno
1 tbsp of olive oil
Half sliced tomato
Some lettuce leaves
Burger buns

NUTRITION FACTS PER SERVES
Calories 98 kcal
Total Fat 2 gm
Total carbohydrates 8 gm
Protein 27 gm

Directions

1. Set the grill on a moderate flame setting.
2. Combine the cheddar cheese, cream cheese, garlic powder, and jalapeno in a bowl.
3. Combine the meat, some onions, salt, and pepper.
4. Take a tiny piece of cream cheese and wrap the meat around it, covering the cheese.
5. With an oil brush, grill each piece of meat
6. Now grill the meat for ten minutes till it is cooked tenderly.
7. Take the buns, put the lettuce leaves, then sliced tomatoes, onion rings, cheese-covered meat, and the jalapeno dressing in the end, and cover with another bun.
8. Make more burgers and serve.

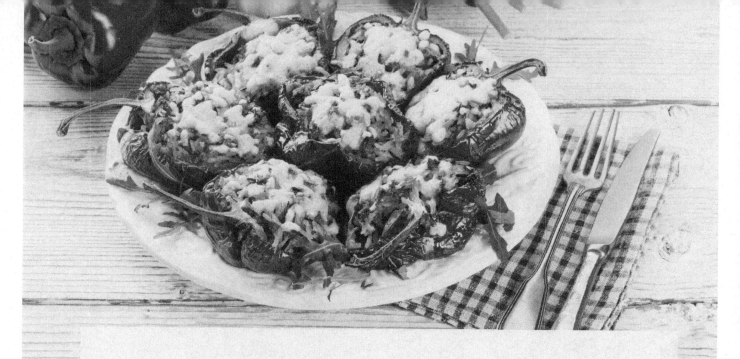

Cheese Stuffed Peppers with Beef

L&G count: 1 lean, 1 green, 1 healthy fat

SERVINGS: 4   PREPPING TIME: 10 MINS   COOKING TIME: 20 MINS

Ingredients

One-pound sweet peppers

20 oz lean beef

8 tbsp salsa

4 tbsp olives

1 tbsp all-purpose seasoning

6 tbsp cream

½ cup cheese

Fresh cilantro

NUTRITION FACTS PER SERVES

Calories 224 kcal

Total Fat 2 gm

Total carbohydrates 9 gm

Protein 38 gm

Directions

1. In a pan, cook meat for eight minutes while adding all-purpose seasoning.
2. Slice pepper into half, then scoops the inside for filling.
3. Start stuffing the peppers with the beef and cheese after giving them a minute in the microwave to soften them.
4. Serving the sweet peppers while the cheese melts under the grill.

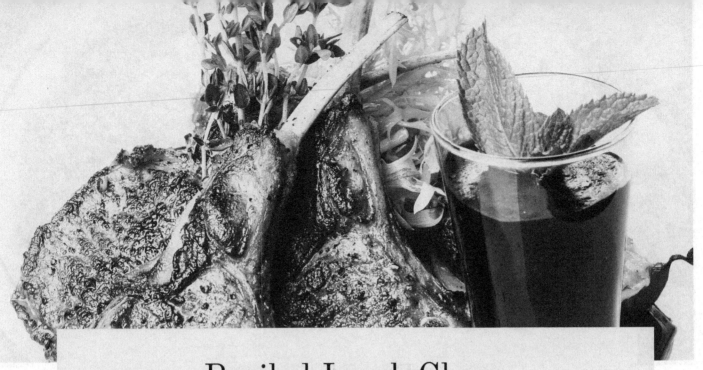

Broiled Lamb Chops

L&G count: 1 leaner, 3 condiments, 1 healthy fat

SERVINGS: 4   PREPPING TIME: 3 MIN   COOKING TIME: 10 MIN

Ingredients

Eight trimmed lamb
chops
½ tsp of salt
½ tsp of black pepper
1 lemon

2 cloves of garlic
2 cups of baby arugula
½ tbsp of olive oil
2 tbsp of water
Cooking spray
1 tbsp of pine nuts

NUTRITION FACTS PER SERVES
Calories 170 kcal
Total Fat 5 gm
Total carbohydrates 8 gm
Protein 24 gm

Directions

1. Spray cooking spray and preheat your oven to broil.
2. Season The lamb with salt & pepper, then put it in the oven.
3. Broil the meat for five minutes on each side.
4. Mix the components inside a mixer till uniform: lemon juice, garlic, lemon peel, pepper, arugula, salt, pine nuts, and water.
5. Serve this sauce with lamb.

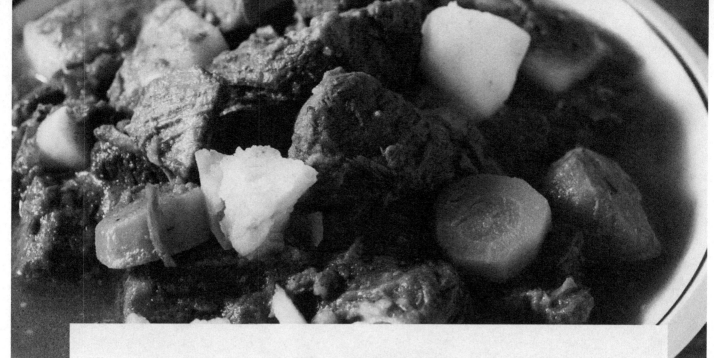

Beef Stew

L&G count: 2 condiments, 2 greens

SERVINGS: 4   PREPPING TIME: 10 MINS   COOKING TIME: 20 MINS

Ingredients

6 ounces diced beef

1 tbsp lime juice

1 tbsp cumin

½ tsp salt

1/2 tsp pepper

1 slice of jicama

8 radishes

½ cup cilantro

4 carrots

NUTRITION FACTS PER SERVES

Calories 200 kcal

Total Fat 9 gm

Total carbohydrates 15 gm

Protein 24 gm

Directions

1. Add olive oil, coriander, cumin, lemon juice, and beef over a moderate flame in a pan and let it cook.

2. Season with salt & pepper as required

3. Serve with jicama, radishes, cilantro, and carrots on top, but before serving, let it simmer on low flame for five minutes.

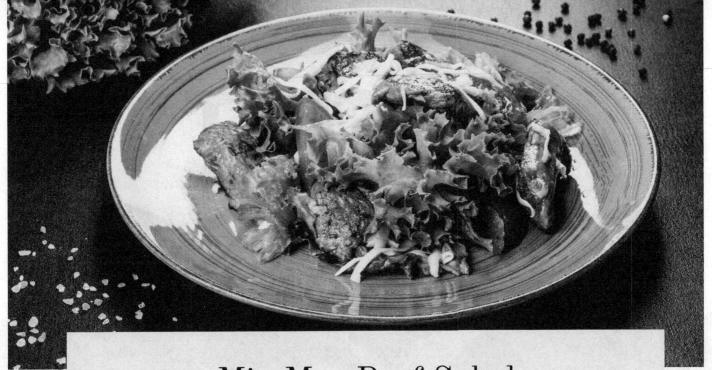

Min Mac Beef Salad

L&G count: 1 lean, 3 condiments, 1 healthy fat, 2 greens

SERVINGS: 1   PREPPING TIME: 5 MINS   COOKING TIME: 10 MINS

Ingredients

Half cup of onions

½ cup lean beef

One tsp of vinegar

Pinch of onion powder

3 cups of romaine lettuce

½ cup of cheddar cheese

2 tomatoes

NUTRITION FACTS PER SERVES

Calories 49 kcal

Total Fat 4 gm

Total carbohydrates 8 gm

Protein 16 gm

Directions

1. Cook onions in a hot, lightly oiled pan for three minutes
2. Brown the beef after adding it to the pan.
3. Add vinegar and onion powder, and stir well.
4. Add cheese and beef mixture over the lettuce.
5. Add pickles and drizzle sauce over it, then serve.

DESSERT
Easy recipes

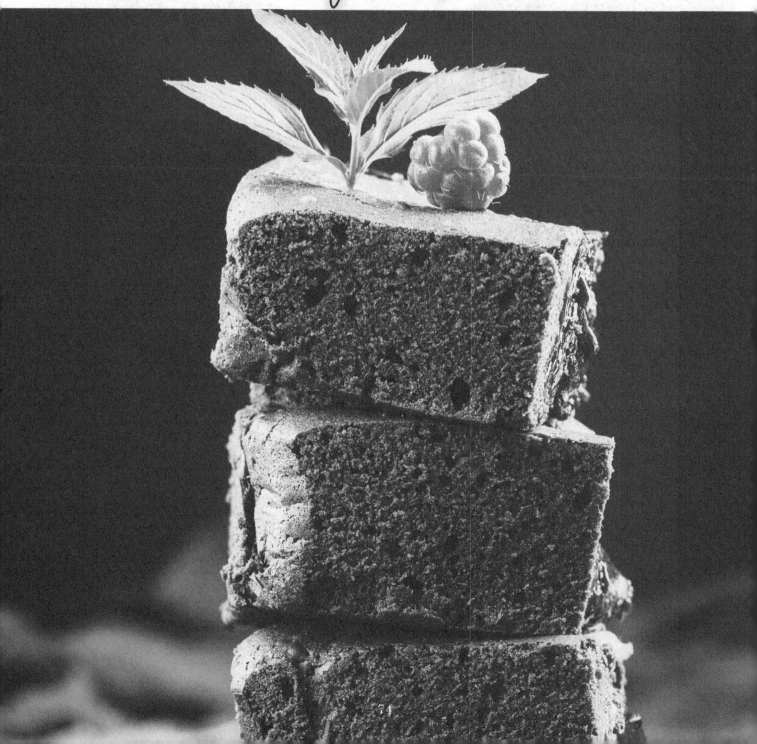

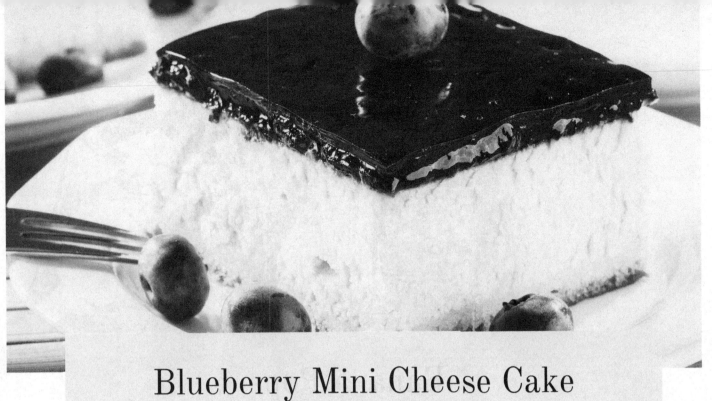

Blueberry Mini Cheese Cake

L&G count: 2 healthy fats, 3 condiments

SERVINGS: 8   PREPPING TIME: 25 MINS   COOKING TIME: 0 MINS

Ingredients

½ cup of cream cheese

28g coconut palm sugar

½ cup of Greek yogurt

Two tbsps. of lemon juice

Two tbsps. of blueberry preserves

½ cup of blueberries

3 tbsp of almonds

4 dates

NUTRITION FACTS PER SERVES

Calories 138 kcal

Total Fat 2 gm

Total carbohydrates 27 gm

Protein 4 gm

Directions

1. Combine the cream cheese, yogurt, sugar, and lemon juice in a medium bowl.
2. Put it in the fridge till ready to use after three minutes of electric hand beating.
3. Combine blueberries and preserves in a different bowl.
4. Add almonds to a food processor and pulse until they resemble crumb consistency.
5. Dates and pulse should be combined.
6. Evenly distribute the almond and date mixture among the servings.
7. Add half of the cheesecake with yogurt batter on top, then a spoonful of the blueberry concoction.
8. Put it in the fridge for three hours in the refrigerator, then serve.

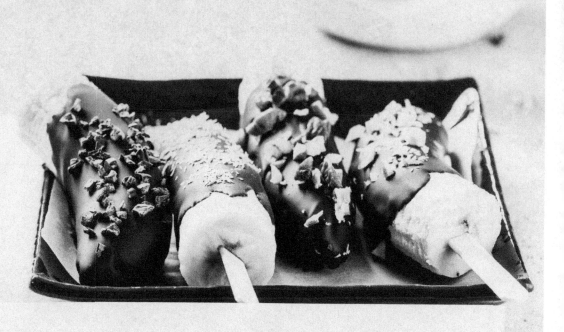

Banana Pops

L&G count: 3 condiments

SERVINGS: 2

PREPPING TIME: 5 MINS

COOKING TIME: 0 MIN

Ingredients

3 bananas

Two tbsps. of cocoa powder

One-Third cup water

Two drops of liquid stevia

One tbsp cocoa powder

One tbsp walnuts

One tbsp coconut flour

NUTRITION FACTS PER SERVES

Calories 241 kcal

Total Fat 1 gm

Total carbohydrates 58 gm

Protein 3 gm

Directions

1. Put a stick inside two bananas.
2. Bananas should be frozen.
3. The remaining bananas, water, cocoa powder, and stevia should combine to make a smooth chocolate syrup.
4. Bananas must be dipped in chocolate.
5. To your liking, garnish with any choice of chopped nuts, coconut flour, or cocoa
6. Then put them in the refrigerator for a while before serving.

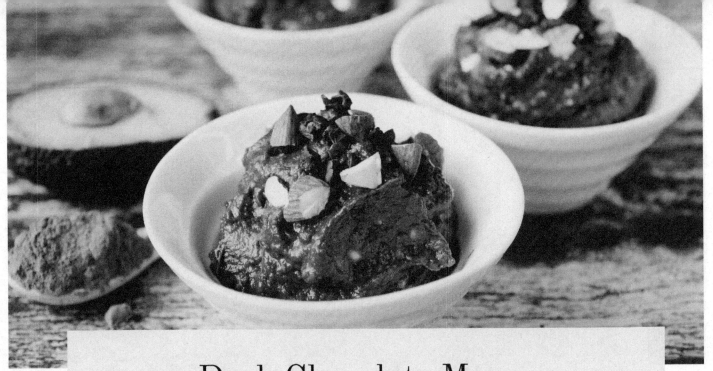

Dark Chocolate Mouse

L&G count: 1/2 healthy fat, 2 condiments, 1 green

SERVINGS: 2   PREPPING TIME: 5 MINS   COOKING TIME: 0 MINS

Ingredients

Two ripe avocados

3 tbsp of dark cocoa powder

One tsp of vanilla

Two tbsp stevia powder

4 tbsps. of almond milk

A pinch of salt

2 tbsp walnuts and almonds

NUTRITION FACTS PER SERVES

Calories 235 kcal

Total Fat 10 gm

Total carbohydrates 12 gm

Protein 8 gm

Directions

1. Blend the items in a food processor till they are well combined.
2. Now pour this mix into serving gasses and let them sit in the fridge for an half an hour or so.
3. Enjoy a chilled serving!

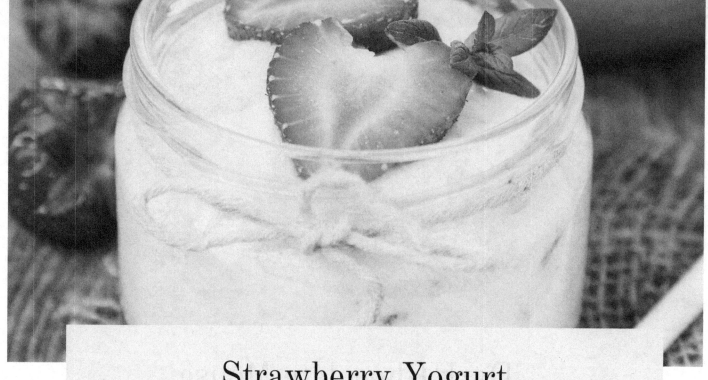

Strawberry Yogurt

L&G count: 1 healthy fat, 1 condiment

SERVINGS: 4   PREPPING TIME: 5 MIN   COOKING TIME: 0 MIN

Ingredients

Half cup of yogurt.
One-Third cup of
strawberry jam

Some fresh strawberry

NUTRITION FACTS PER SERVES
Calories 207 kcal
Total Fat 1 gm
Total carbohydrates 46 gm
Protein 5 gm

Directions

1. Combine the entire components and refrigerate.
2. For extra flavor, add strawberry chunks and enjoy!

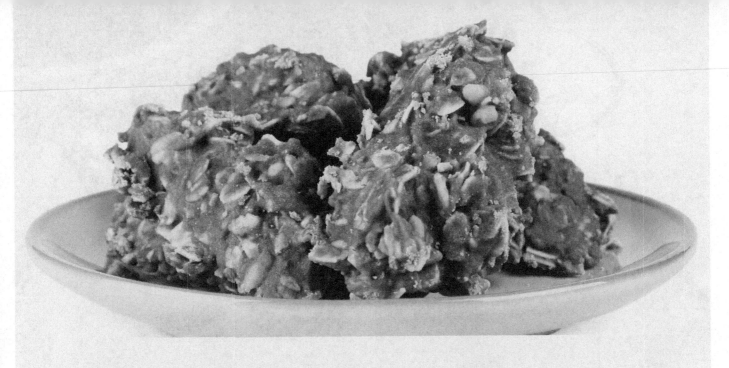

Frozen Yogurt Bites

L&G count: 1 healthy fat, 1 condiment

SERVINGS: 3   PREPPING TIME: 10 MINS   COOKING TIME: 0 MINS

Ingredients

Two-Third cup of Greek yogurt

½ cup of granola

3 tbsps. of chocolate chips

NUTRITION FACTS PER SERVES

Calories 180 kcal

Total Fat 2 gm

Total carbohydrates 19 gm

Protein 24 gm

Directions

1. Combine yogurt and granola in a bowl.
2. Place a portion of the mixture in an ice cube tray and then freeze till they become solid.
3. Take out of the tray, then cover frozen cubes with melted chocolate.
4. Once more, freeze until solid, then eat!

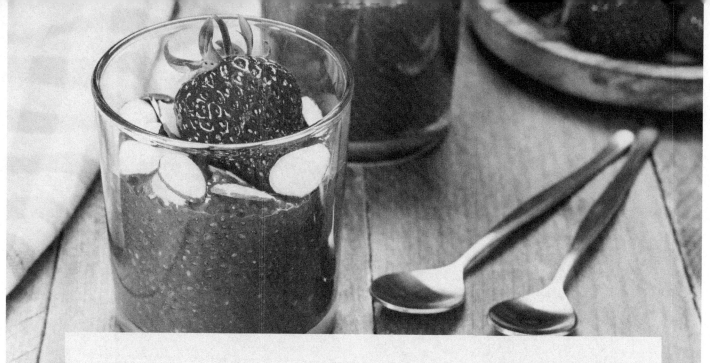

Chocolate Pudding with Chia Seed

L&G count: 2 healthy fats, 2 condiments

SERVINGS: 4   PREPPING TIME: 10 MINS   COOKING TIME: 0 MINS

Ingredients

Two cups of almond milk

Four tbsps of chia seeds

Two tbsps of almond butter

Two tbsps of cocoa powder

4 large dates

1 tsp of vanilla extract

strawberries and slivered almonds to decorate

NUTRITION FACTS PER SERVES

Calories 219 kcal

Total Fat 7 gm

Total carbohydrates 19 gm

Protein 12 gm

Directions

1. Mix the entire components inside a container & stir.
2. Keep cold for three to four hours.
3. Blend the mixture in a blender till it's smooth.
4. Add more fruits or nuts as a garnish and serve.

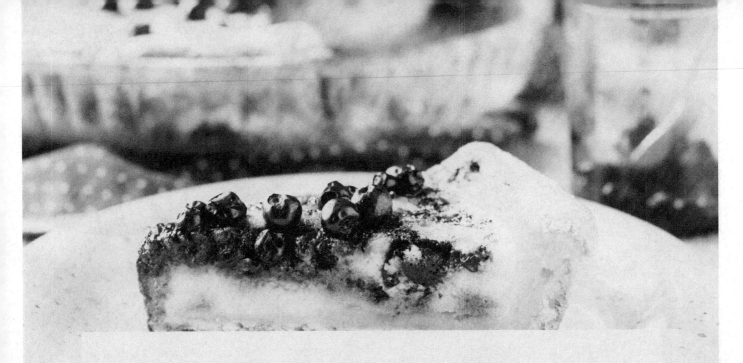

Berry Yogurt Bake

L&G count: 1 healthy fat, 3 condiments

SERVINGS: 4   PREPPING TIME: 15 MINS   COOKING TIME: 30 MINS

Ingredients

4 large size beaten eggs

½ tsp of vanilla extract

One tbsp of corn flour

Three tbsps of honey

One cup of Greek yogurt

1 cup of blueberries

Icing sugar for garnish

NUTRITION FACTS PER SERVES

Calories 105 kcal

Total Fat 9 gm

Total carbohydrates 28 gm

Protein 11 gm

Directions

1. To form a smooth mixture, combine corn flour, eggs, yogurt, and honey in a bowl.
2. Set the oven to 350°F.
3. Spread half the berries with the yogurt mixture on a baking dish.
4. Add the other left berries on top, then bake for 20 minutes.
5. Use sugar to dust and then serve.

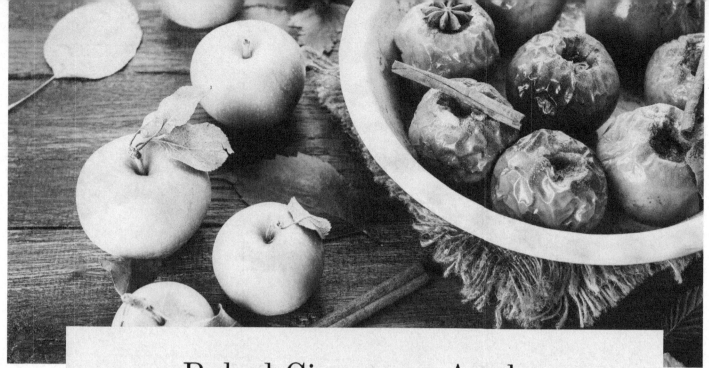

Baked Cinnamon Apples

L&G count: 1 green, 2 condiments

SERVINGS: 2   PREPPING TIME: 5 MINS   COOKING TIME: 20 MINS

Ingredients

6 green apples

½ cup of melted butter

½ teaspoon of apple pie spice

Half tsp of cinnamon

Half cup star anise

3 packets of raw stevia

NUTRITION FACTS PER SERVES

Calories 150 kcal

Total Fat 4 gm

Total carbohydrates 53 gm

Protein 1 gm

Directions

1. Turn the temperature of the oven to 356 °F.
2. The baking paper should be used to line a baking sheet.
3. Add the melted butter to the baking dish with the cleaned apples.
4. Combine the cinnamon, stevia, apple pie spice, star anise, and salt in a bowl.
5. The mixture should be poured over the apples, then covered with foil.
6. For twenty minutes, bake while covered.
7. Bake for the next fifteen min without the lid. Serve hot.
8. Just a few cinnamon sticks might be used as a garnish.

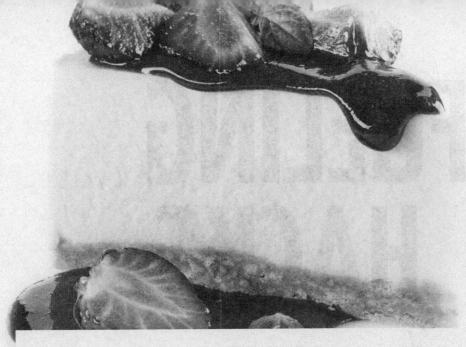
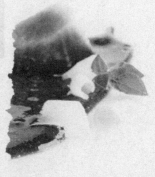

Strawberry Cake

L&G count: 2 healthy fats, 3 condiments

SERVINGS: 8   PREPPING TIME: 25 MIN   COOKING TIME: 0 MIN

Ingredients

Half cup of cream cheese

2 tbsp of coconut palm sugar

½ cup of Greek yogurt

Two tbsps. of lemon juice

Two tbsps of strawberry preserves

½ cup of diced strawberries

3 tbsp of whole almonds

4 dates

NUTRITION FACTS PER SERVES

Calories 138 kcal

Total Fat 2 gm

Total carbohydrates 27 gm

Protein 4 gm

Directions

1. Combine the cream cheese, yogurt, sugar, and lemon juice in a medium bowl.

2. Refrigerate till ready to use after three minutes of electric hand beating.

3. Combine strawberries and preserves in a different bowl.

4. Add almonds to a food processor and pulse until they resemble crumb consistency.

5. Dates and pulse should be combined.

6. Evenly distribute the almond and date mixture among the servings.

7. Place half of the cheesecake batter on top, followed by the yogurt and strawberry combination.

8. After three hours in the refrigerator, serve.

FUELING HACKS
Easy recipes

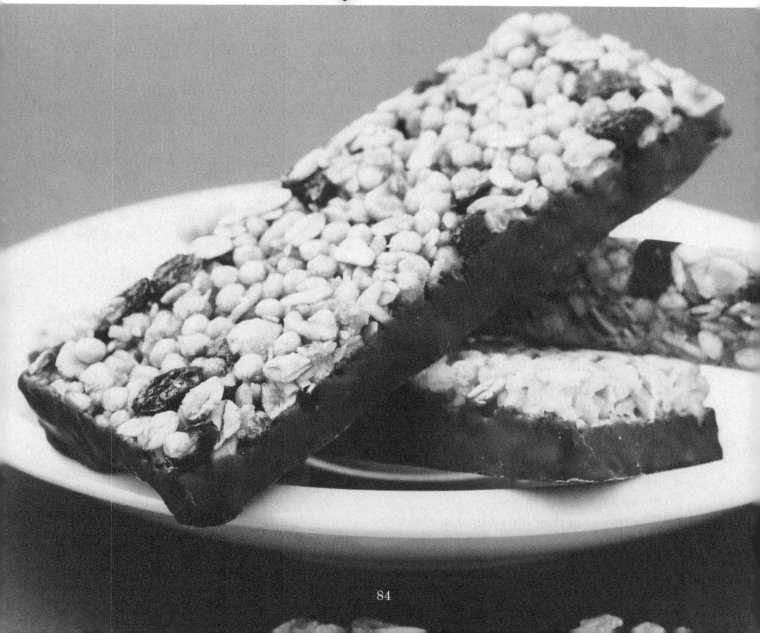

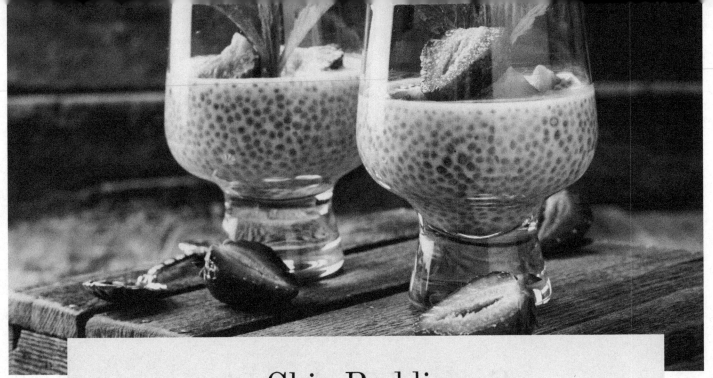

Chia Pudding

L&G count: 1 fueling, 2 healthy fats, 2 condiments

SERVINGS: 2   PREPPING TIME: 5 MINS   COOKING TIME: 0 MINS

Ingredients

One packet of chia
smoothie powder

¼ cup chia seeds

1 cup coconut milk

½ tsp lemon zest

4 sliced strawberries

NUTRITION FACTS PER SERVES

Calories 82 kcal

Total Fat 7 gm

Total carbohydrates 11 gm

Protein 13 gm

Directions

1. Put every ingredient in a bowl except the strawberries.
2. Stir them well, and then chill the mixture overnight in a fridge.
3. Serve the dish with half-sliced strawberries.

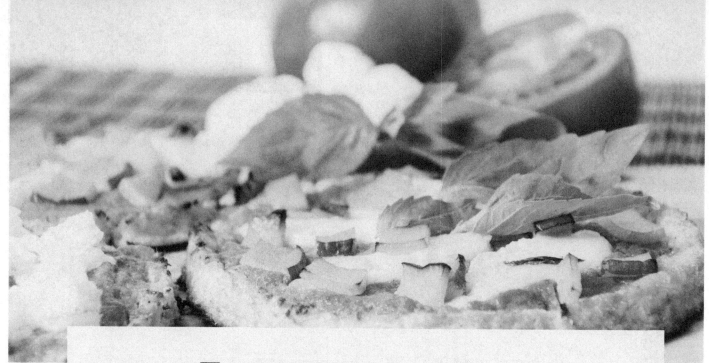

Egg and Turkey Pizza

L&G count: 1 fueling, 1 green, 1 condiment

SERVINGS: 2   PREPPING TIME: 10 MINS   COOKING TIME: 35 MINS

Ingredients

One and a half cups
mozzarella cheese

Two eggs

3 tbsp parmesan cheese

Salt and Italian seasoning

6 slices of turkey rump

1 tbsp onions

A few basil leaves

NUTRITION FACTS PER SERVES

Calories 217 kcal

Total Fat 12 gm

Total carbohydrates 16 gm

Protein 35 gm

Directions

1. The oven temperature is set to 375 °F
2. Half of the cheese, Parmesan, salt, plus Italian seasoning should be combined with eggs.
3. This mixture should be spooned into 12 molds, compressed using your fingers to create a thin crust, then bake for twenty minutes.
4. The remaining cheese, onion, and turkey rump should be sprinkled on top. Bake till the cheese melts. Use basil leaves as decoration.

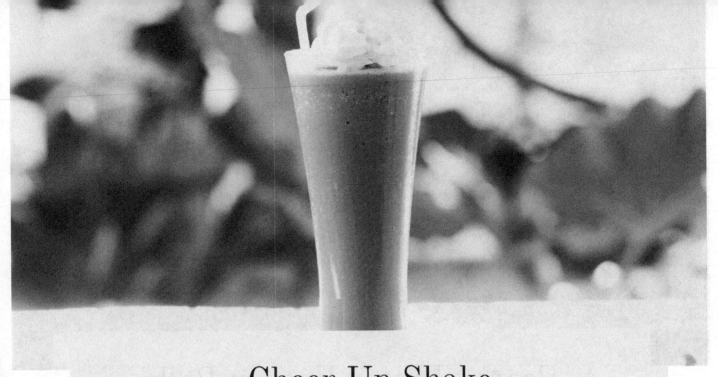

Cheer Up Shake

L&G count: 1 fueling, ½ leaner, 2 ½ condiments

SERVINGS: 1   PREPPING TIME: 5 MINS   COOKING TIME: 0 MINS

Ingredients

1 pack of coffee powder

½ cup ice

6-ounce yogurt

½ cup almond milk

2 tbsp chocolate syrup

·Whipped cream

NUTRITION FACTS PER SERVES

Calories 99 kcal

Total Fat 9 gm

Total carbohydrates 5 gm

Protein 8 gm

Directions

1. Blend the first four ingredients thoroughly in a blender.
2. Add cream and chocolate syrup on the top of the drink after pouring the mix into the serving glass.
3. It will help boost weight loss and provide energy for the body.

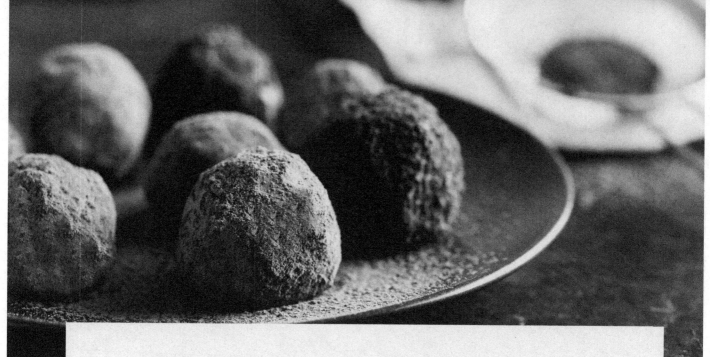

Peanut Butter Energy Balls

L&G count: 1 fueling

SERVINGS: 1   PREPPING TIME: 5 MINS   COOKING TIME: 0 MINS

Ingredients

Two peanut butter bars   4 oz of dry cookies

One tbsp peanut butter   1 tbsp water
powder
                                1 tbsp of chocolate

NUTRITION FACTS PER SERVES

Calories 124 kcal

Total Fat 12 gm

Total carbohydrates 5 gm

Protein 30 gm

Directions

1. Mix the water and powdered peanut butter in a bowl to create a little thick paste.
2. They will become softer by baking the peanut butter bars for thirty seconds.
3. Form a dough by combining the paste and the softened bar.
4. Make little balls next using your hands or a scoop.
5. Keep them chilled in a fridge till they're ready to be served.

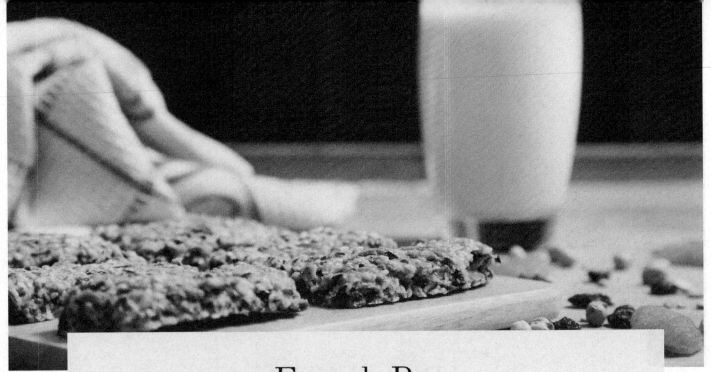

French Bars

L&G count: 3 condiments

SERVINGS: 2   PREPPING TIME: 15 MINS   COOKING TIME: 5 MINS

Ingredients

Two cups cereal

2 tbsp low-fat cheese

6 tbsp egg white only

1 cup dry fruits of your choice

Cooking spray

NUTRITION FACTS PER SERVES

Calories 194 kcal

Total Fat 21 gm

Total carbohydrates 11 gm

Protein 39 gm

Directions

1. In a blender, combine the cereals with the cheese and egg white to produce dough.
2. Using this dough, create 6 lengthy bars.
3. Take a pan and spritz the cooking spray in it.
4. In a pan, cook these bars until golden brown on both sides.
5. Serve the bars with an energy drink.

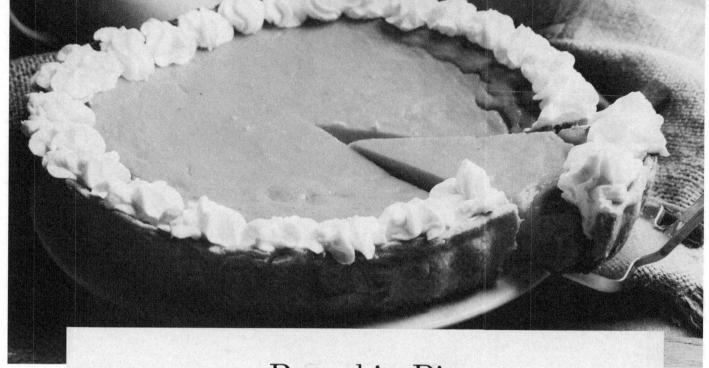

Pumpkin Pie

L&G count: 1 fueling, 1 condiment

SERVINGS:1   PREPPING TIME: 5 MINS   COOKING TIME: 0 MINS

Ingredients

One piece gingerbread

4 ounce almond milk

4 ounce brewed coffee

½ cup ice

One-Eighth cup pumpkin pie filling

2 tbsp whipped cream

NUTRITION FACTS PER SERVES

Calories 116 kcal

Total Fat 6 gm

Total carbohydrates 3gm

Protein 29 gm

Directions

1. Blend all the ingredients except the whipped cream.
2. Blend until it gets smooth, then put it in a dish and set it in the fridge for a while.
3. Then top with cream and serve the pie after cutting it into pieces.

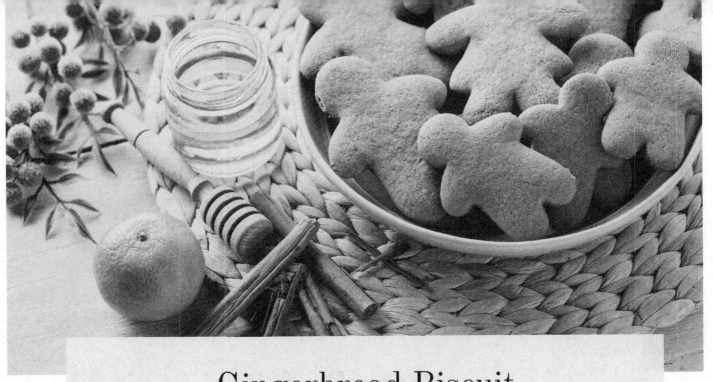

Gingerbread Biscuit

L&G count: 1 fueling, 1condiment

SERVINGS:4   PREPPING TIME: 5 MINS   COOKING TIME: 55 MINS

Ingredients

One packet gingerbread

¼ tsp baking powder

2 eggs whites

2 tbsp Maple syrup

·Cooking spray

NUTRITION FACTS PER SERVES

Calories 67 kcal

Total Fat 1 gm

Total carbohydrates 9 gm

Protein 10 gm

Directions

1. Warm the oven to 350 °F

2. Open the gingerbread sachet inside a container

3. Combine baking powder & egg white in a bowl to form a dough.

4. Put the dough for the biscuits onto a baking sheet using a spoon or some other utensil.

5. Put them aside, covered for half an hour.

6. The biscuits must be One inch thick when cut diagonally. Place the cut piece down on the paper and bake for fifteen minutes. After that, remove it and allow it to cool.

7. When chilled, serve.

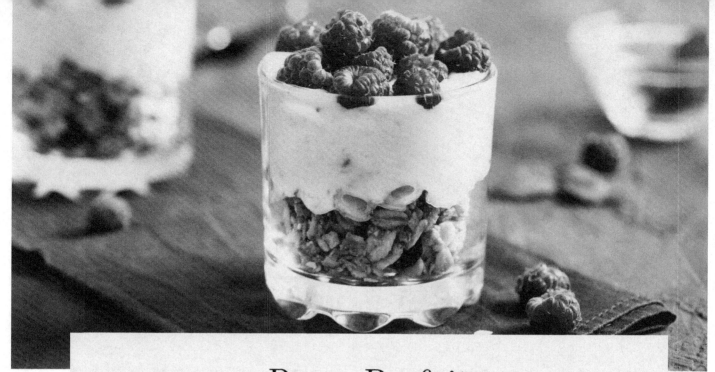

Berry Parfait

L&G count: ½ fueling, ½ leanest, 2 healthy fats, 3 condiments

SERVINGS: 2   PREPPING TIME: 5 MINS   COOKING TIME: 0 MINS

Ingredients

1 ½ cups yogurt

¼ cup strawberry cream cheese

1 cup sugar

¼ cup granola

Two-Third ounce almonds

1 cup raspberries

NUTRITION FACTS PER SERVES
Calories 85 kcal
Total Fat 3 gm
Total carbohydrates 7 gm
Protein 10 gm

Directions

1. For two minutes, Blend everything in a blender, except the yogurt and cream cheese. Save some raspberries for decoration.

2. Combine the yogurt and strawberry cream cheese in a bowl.

3. Put the granola inside the bottom of a serving glass, then top it with the yogurt, cream cheese, and raspberries.

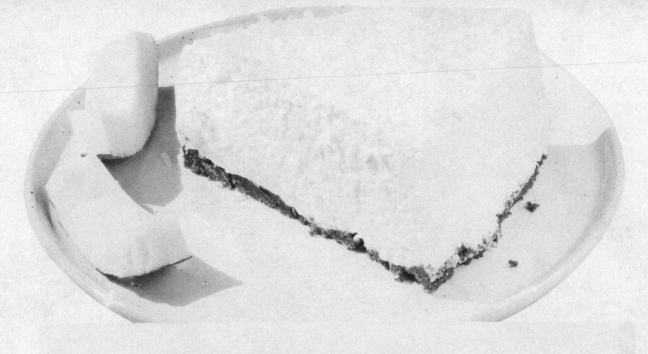

Coconut Pie

L&G count: 1 fueling, ¼ leaner, 1 healthy fat, 1 ½ condiments

SERVINGS: 2   PREPPING TIME: 30 MINS   COOKING TIME: 0 MINS

Ingredients

1 chocolate bar

One cup cream cheese pudding

½ cup almond milk

Cooking spray

2 tbsp whipped cream

·1 ½ cups coconuts

NUTRITION FACTS PER SERVES

Calories 100 kcal

Total Fat 5 gm

Total carbohydrates 3 gm

Protein 7 gm

Directions

1. Put the chocolate bar in the ramekin and warm it just enough to melt it.
2. Then combine pudding and milk, and add it to the chocolate in the ramekin.
3. Let it chill for 30 minutes in the refrigerator.
4. Add whipped cream and coconut flakes over the to

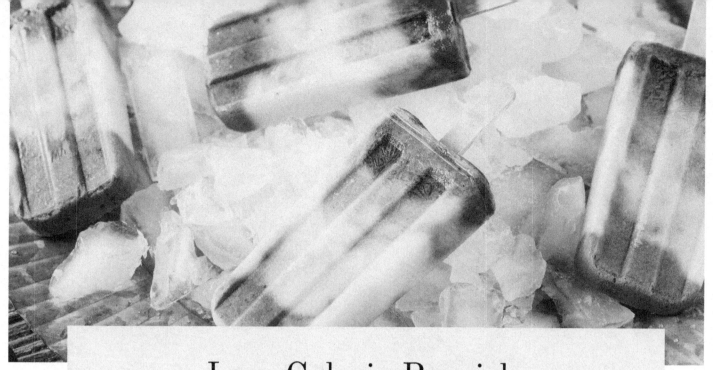

Low-Calorie Popsicle

L&G count: ½ fueling, ¼ leaner, ½ condiment

SERVINGS:6   PREPPING TIME: 25 MINS   COOKING TIME: 0 MINS

Ingredients

1 cup vanilla almond
milk

2 cups yogurt

1 packet of mint
smoothie powder

1 packet of strawberry
smoothie powder

1 packet of vanilla
milkshake powder

1 cup of sugar

NUTRITION FACTS PER SERVES

Calories 187 kcal

Total Fat 8 gm

Total carbohydrates 19 gm

Protein 34 gm

Directions

1. Blend milk, yogurt, and sugar with 1 packet of mint smoothie powder.
2. This liquid should be poured into the Popsicle molds and frozen overnight.
3. Use the same procedure for the vanilla and strawberry shakes and additional flavors.
4. Or you can create one Popsicle with three distinct layers.

Honey Oats Baked

L&G count: 1 fueling, 1 healthy fat, 1 condiment

SERVINGS: 4   PREPPING TIME: 5 MINS   COOKING TIME: 25 MINS

Ingredients

4 cups honey oats

3 tbsps egg white

½ tsp baking powder

1 cup almond milk

1 ½ ounce walnuts

One and half ounce almonds

One cup raisins

Cooking spray

¼ tsp cinnamon

NUTRITION FACTS PER SERVES

Calories 101 kcal

Total Fat 1 gm

Total carbohydrates 19 gm

Protein 30 gm

Directions

1. The oven should be heated to 350 degrees Fahrenheit
2. Inside a container, mix the oats, milk, egg white, and baking powder. Stir well until the egg white is completely incorporated.
3. Finally, fill 4 containers with this mixture, leaving 1.5 inches of space at the top.
4. Bake it for twenty minutes till the top is golden.
5. Now garnish cinnamon on top.

After letting it cool, utilize it within five days of production while keeping it chilled.

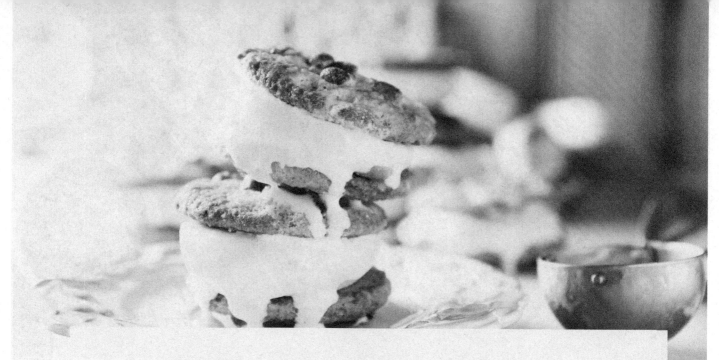

Lemon Sandwich Cookies

L&G count: 1 fueling, 1 leaner

SERVINGS: 2   PREPPING TIME: 10 MINS   COOKING TIME: 3 MINS

Ingredients

Two lemon crisp bars

One and a half cups yogurt

One ounce lemon gelatin

NUTRITION FACTS PER SERVES

Calories 34 kcal

Total Fat 3 gm

Total carbohydrates 5 gm

Protein 8 gm

Directions

1. Break the two bars into six pieces, place them in the six slots of a microwave-safe cupcake pan, and microwave for thirty seconds.
2. Mix the lemon gelatin with yogurt and microwave it for two minutes
3. Fill the 6 spaces with a mixture of yogurt and let it sit in the fridge.
4. When it is cooled and becomes rigid, serve.

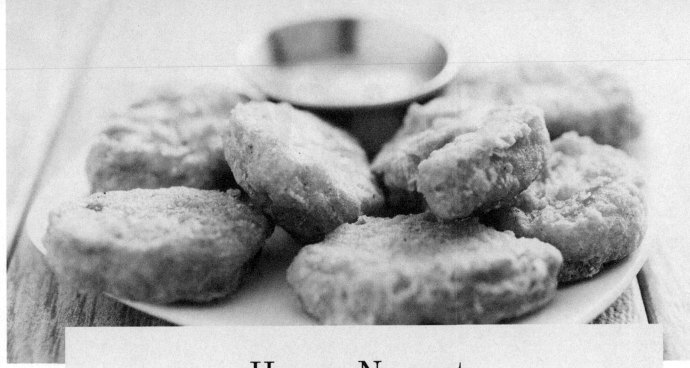

Honey Nuggets

L&G count: 1 fueling, 1 leaner, 2 condiments

SERVINGS: 2   PREPPING TIME: 5 MINS   COOKING TIME: 20 MINS

Ingredients

12-ounce chicken

1 egg

2 tbsp onion powder

2 tbsp mustard powder

¼ cup yogurt

2 tbsp mustard

Cooking spray

¼ tsp garlic powder

NUTRITION FACTS PER SERVES

Calories 224 kcal

Total Fat 9 gm

Total carbohydrates 9 gm

Protein 28 gm

Directions

1. Warm up the oven to 375 degrees Fahrenheit

2. Put the egg and the finely diced onions in another bowl.

3. Take the chicken and cover it with onion as well as mustard powder after dipping it in the egg.

4. Place cooking spray on the chicken on a baking pan. Set the oven to 302 °F, then bake for twenty minutes.

5. Prepare the yogurt with spicy mustard, garlic powder, and croquettes.

6. Serve with yogurt with spicy mustard, garlic powder, and croquettes.

SNACKS

Easy recipes

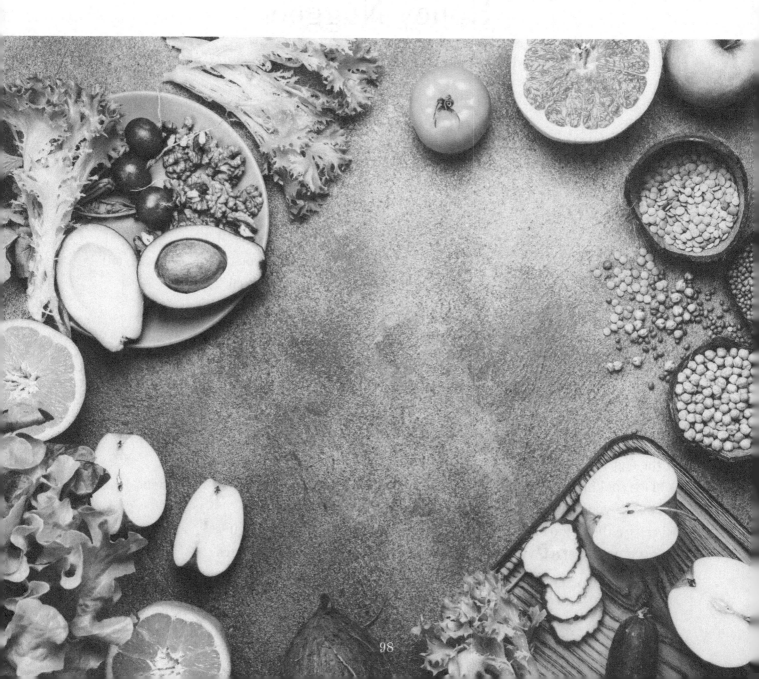

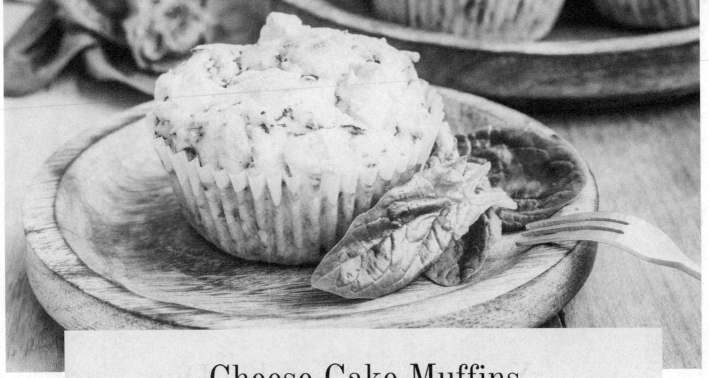

Cheese Cake Muffins

L&G count: 1 healthy fat, 2 condiments

SERVINGS: 4   PREPPING TIME: 10 MINS   COOKING TIME: 0 MINS

Ingredients

1 ½ cups of Greek yogurt

2 tbsp of pudding mix

½ tsp of peppermint extract

Mint leaves

1 pack of cookie bars

NUTRITION FACTS PER SERVES

Calories 90 kcal

Total Fat 4 gm

Total carbohydrates 11 gm

Protein 1 gm

Directions

1. Use a cupcake liner to line a muffin pan.

2. The cookie bars should be cut in half and crunched in the microwave.

3. Microwave them for twenty-five minutes, then take them out.

4. The mix of Greek yogurt, sugar, and pudding should be thoroughly combined with the microwaved cookie bars.

5. On the muffin liners, evenly distribute the mixture.

6. Put the muffin pan in the freezer for almost half an hour.

·Add mint leaves on top and serve.

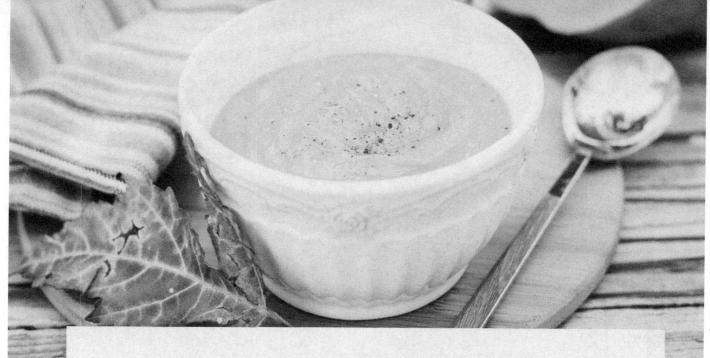

Yogurt and Pumpkin Dip

L&G count: 1 healthy fat, 2 condiments

SERVINGS: 5   PREPPING TIME: 5 MINS   COOKING TIME: 0 MINS

Ingredients

One cup of yogurt

½ cup of pumpkin puree

1 tsp of cinnamon

One tsp of vanilla extract

½ tsp of ginger

1 tsp of maple syrup

NUTRITION FACTS PER SERVES

Calories 48 kcal

Total Fat 0 gm

Total carbohydrates 8 gm

Protein 3 gm

Directions

1. Mix the entire components in a container
2. Combine everything all together.
3. Then serve with your favorite food.

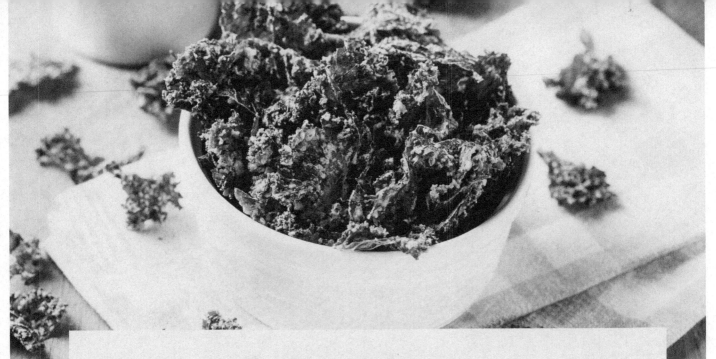

Kale Chips

L&G count: 1 green, 1 condiment

SERVINGS: 3   PREPPING TIME: 5 MINS   COOKING TIME: 15 MINS

Ingredients

One and a half cups
kale leaves
Cooking spray

½ tsp of sea salt

NUTRITION FACTS PER SERVES

Calories 100 kcal

Total Fat 0 gm

Total carbohydrates 15 gm

Protein 5 gm

Directions

1. Blend the entire components inside a container
2. Combine well and then serve.

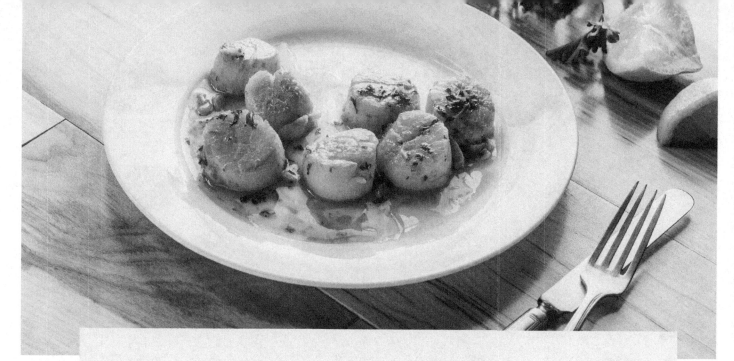

Caramel Scallops

L&G count: 1 lean, 2 healthy fats

SERVINGS: 4   PREPPING TIME: 5 MINS   COOKING TIME: 10 MINS

Ingredients

1 ¾ scallops

2 tbsps lemon oil

Half cup chicken broth

Four tbsps balsamic vinegar

·Some garlic leaves

NUTRITION FACTS PER SERVES

Calories 112 kcal

Total Fat 2 gm

Total carbohydrates 9 gm

Protein 18 gm

Directions

1. Warm the oil inside a big pot until it sizzles across a moderate flame.

2. Beginning with one at once, place the scallops flat-side down in the pan.

3. Scallops should be cooked for four minutes on moderate flame till they are caramelized.

4. Then flip, and cook the other side for a minute.

5. Add the broth with the vinegar to the pan and let it simmer.

6. Scrape the entire browned bits from the lower part of the pan to deglaze it.

7. Simmer the liquid until it has been cut in half.

8. Garnish with a few garlic leaves before serving.

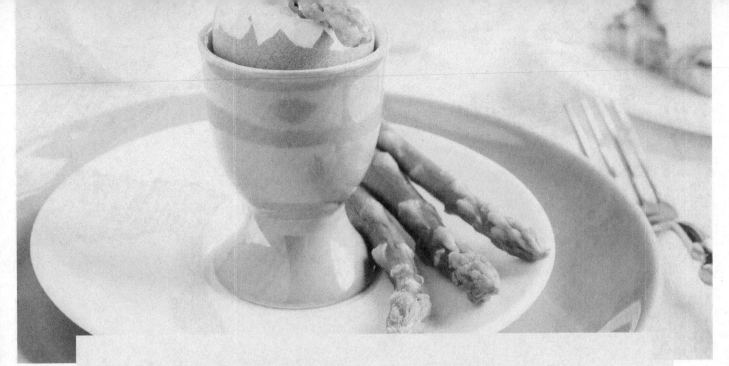

Eggs with Asparagus

L&G count: 1 green, 1 condiment

SERVINGS: 2   PREPPING TIME: 2 MINS   COOKING TIME: 5 MINS

Ingredients

Two soft boil eggs   14 spears of asparagus

NUTRITION FACTS PER SERVES

Calories 103 kcal

Total Fat 6 gm

Total carbohydrates 1 gm

Protein 11 gm

Directions

1. Cut the eggs into half.
2. Steam the asparagus.
3. Serve it with the eggs on a platter.

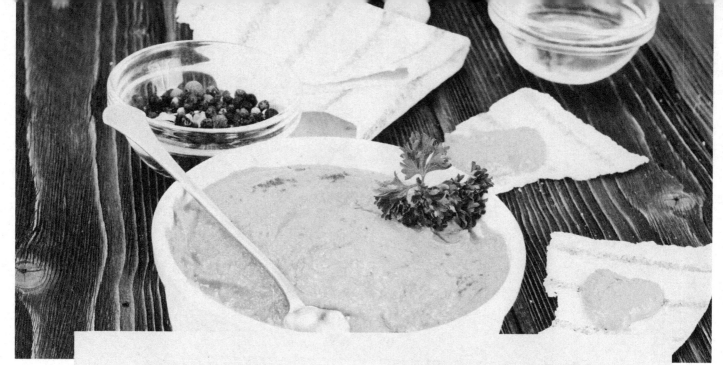

Red Pepper and Chick Pea Dip

L&G count: 3 condiments

SERVINGS: 4   PREPPING TIME: 5 MINS   COOKING TIME: O MINS

Ingredients

One and a half cup
chickpeas
1 garlic clove
Juice of one lemon
2 red peppers

Fresh coriander
4 tbsp olive oil
Pitta bread

NUTRITION FACTS PER SERVES
Calories 200 kcal
Total Fat 2 gm
Total carbohydrates 12 gm
Protein 5 gm

Directions

1. Add chickpeas, olive oil, lemon juice, coriander, garlic, and red peppers to a food processor.
2. Blend well to create a paste, then take it out in a bowl.
3. Toast the pita bread a little.
4. Pair with warm pita bread and serve.

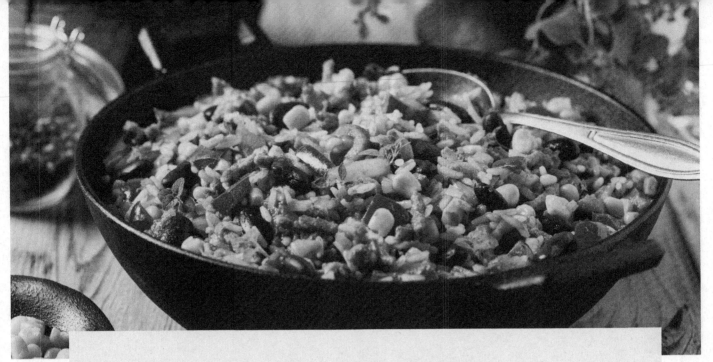

Protein Pot

L&G count: 2 condiments, 1 lean

SERVINGS: 2   PREPPING TIME: 10 MINS   COOKING TIME: 1 MINS

Ingredients

One-third cup lentils

½ cup cherry tomatoes

½ cup cooked chicken
breast pieces

Fresh coriander

4 tbsp of tzatziki

NUTRITION FACTS PER SERVES

Calories 230 kcal

Total Fat 1 gm

Total carbohydrates 12 gm

Protein 7 gm

Directions

1. Lentils should be heated on a high flame in a pan for one minute.
2. Then, leave them to cool for a minute.
3. Make a layer with the lentils, then put chicken, tomatoes, coriander, and tzatziki on top.
4. It is ready to be served.

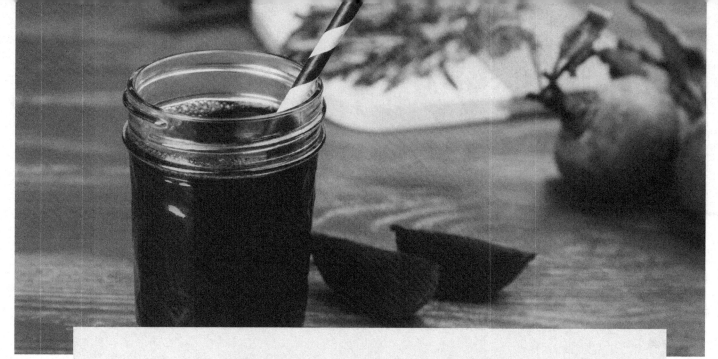

Beet Fruit Dipping

L&G count: 2 condiments, 1 healthy fat

SERVINGS: 4   PREPPING TIME: 10 MINS   COOKING TIME: O MINS

Ingredients

One cup of beetroot   1 Lemon juice

½ teaspoon of cumin   Nigella seeds

One tbsp of mint leaves   3 tbsp of cream

NUTRITION FACTS PER SERVES

Calories 48 kcal

Total Fat 2 gm

Total carbohydrates 6 gm

Protein 2 gm

Directions

1. Cumin and beets should be processed in a food blender till it turns smooth.
2. Add it to a bowl with chopped mint leaves and lemon juice.
3. Mix in the cream.
4. Mint leaves and nigella seeds should be added as a garnish at the end.

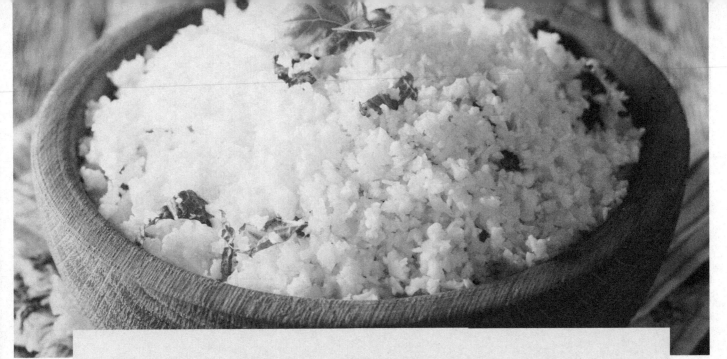

Riced Cauliflower

L&G count: 1 green

SERVINGS: 2   PREPPING TIME: 5 MINS   COOKING TIME: 10 MINS

Ingredients

Two cauliflowers

One teaspoon all-purpose seasoning

Some basil leaves

NUTRITION FACTS PER SERVES

Calories 198 kcal

Total Fat 8 gm

Total carbohydrates 27 gm

Protein 48 gm

Directions

1. The cauliflower should be microwaved tilt so it becomes soft and crisp.
2. Put the cooked cauliflower with the seasoning in a food processor.
3. On high speed, blend cauliflower for about two minutes till it closely resembles rice.
4. Serve with basil leaves as a garnish.

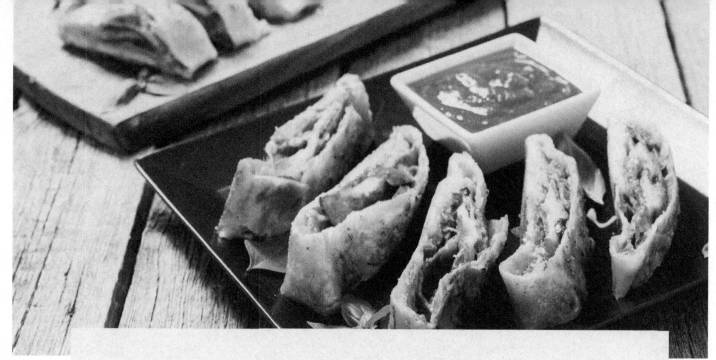

Pepperoni Roll

L&G count: 1 condiment, 2 healthy fats

SERVINGS: 6   PREPPING TIME: 5 MINS   COOKING TIME: 20 MINS

Ingredients

Two cups Pizza sauce

Pizza dough

2 cup Pepperoni

2 cup Mozzarella cheese

½ cup Salted butter

NUTRITION FACTS PER SERVES

Calories 187 kcal

Total Fat 2 gm

Total carbohydrates 4 gm

Protein 23 gm

Directions

1. Get your brick oven ready.
2. Create a skinny, long rectangle using the dough.
3. Pizza sauce, pepperoni, and mozzarella cheese should be spread on the crust.
4. Roll tightly to form a single, incredibly long, thick roll.
5. Cut with a sharp knife into one 1/2-inch slice.
6. Cook pepperoni rolls in a hot oven for almost twenty minutes till the top turns golden brown.
7. Pizza sauce could also be served as dipping.

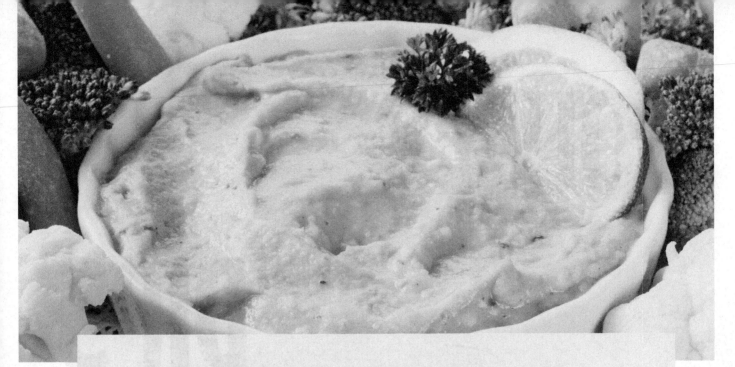

Baked Vegetable Hummus

SERVINGS: 4   PREPPING TIME: 10 MINS   COOKING TIME: 30 MINS

Ingredients

One cup of clumped cauliflower

One cup chopped carrot

1 cup of clumped broccoli

1 tablespoon olive oil

Juice of one lemon

Salt & pepper as required

NUTRITION FACTS PER SERVES

Calories 187 kcal

Total Fat 2 gm

Total carbohydrates 4 gm

Protein 23 gm

Directions

1. Warm up the oven to 356 °F
2. Put vegetables onto a nonstick baking tray, spray with oil, and bake for 30 minutes.
3. Blend the vegetables and other ingredients until smooth.
4. Add water, if necessary, to soften the mixture
5. Enjoy

SOUCES

&

DIPS

Easy recipes

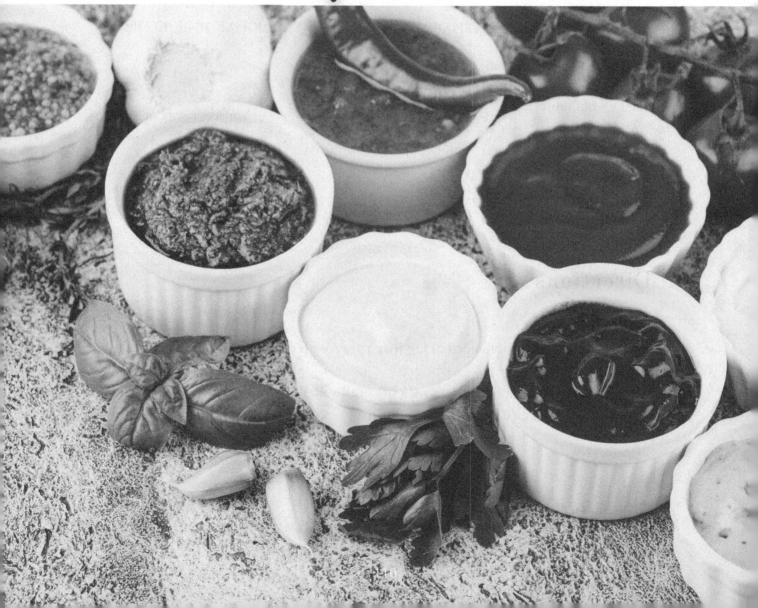

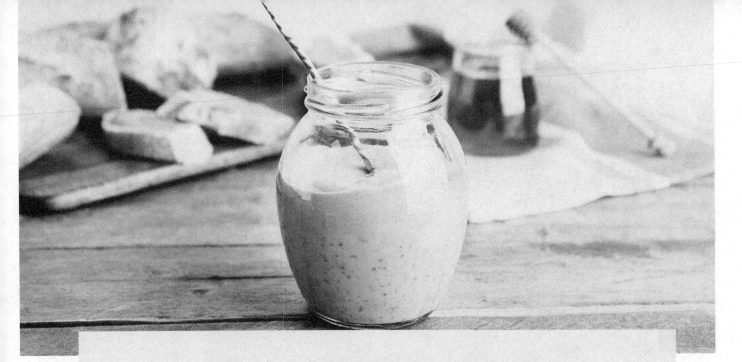

Honey Mustard Sauce

L&G count: 1 condiment

SERVINGS: 6   PREPPING TIME: 10 MINS   COOKING TIME: 10 MINS

Ingredients

Quarter cup honey mustard

¼ cup mayonnaise

½ tsp apple vinegar

¼ tsp all-purpose seasoning

NUTRITION FACTS PER SERVES

Calories 101 kcal

Total Fat 4 gm

Total carbohydrates 7 gm

Protein 11 gm

Directions

1. Add the entire components to a container, combine thoroughly, refrigerate, and use it with any food.

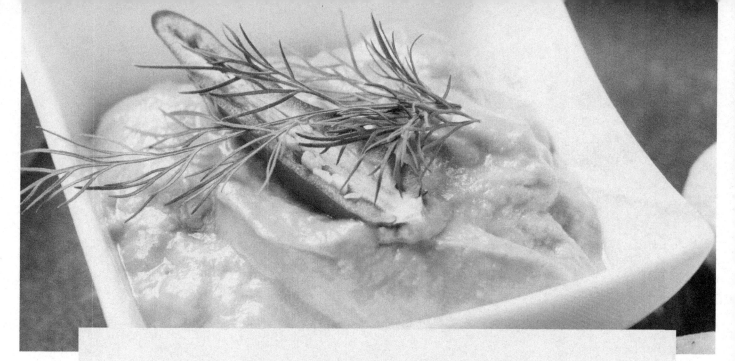

Red Pepper Sauce

L&G count: 1 condiment

SERVINGS: 20   PREPPING TIME: 10 MINS   COOKING TIME: 30 MINS

Ingredients

14 ounces red pepper

1 tbsp all-purpose seasoning

1 tbsp balsamic vinegar

½ tsp apple vinegar

¼ tsp all-purpose seasoning

NUTRITION FACTS PER SERVES

Calories 56 kcal

Total Fat 0 gm

Total carbohydrates 2 gm

Protein 3 gm

Directions

1. Roast the peppers in the oven for 30 minutes at 356 °F
2. Be sure to dry them with a paper towel and skin them
3. Place them in the blender and add the seasoning and balsamic vinegar, mix well, and store in the refrigerator to garnish later with your favorite food.

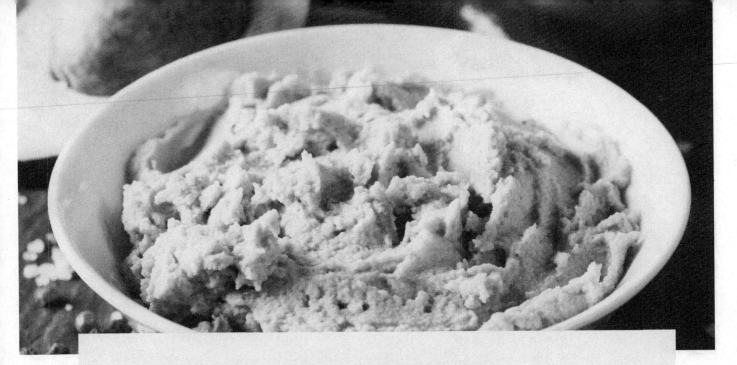

Avocado Dip

L&G count: 1 healthy fat

SERVINGS: 6   PREPPING TIME: 5 MINS   COOKING TIME: 0 MINS

Ingredients

3 avocadoes
All-purpose seasoning

Powdered orange
seasoning
lemon peel seasoning

NUTRITION FACTS PER SERVES

Calories 60 kcal

Total Fat 1 gm

Total carbohydrates 2 gm

Protein 16 gm

Directions

1. Slice the avocado in half, discard the pit, then take out all the avocado using a spoon.
2. Then put it in the bowl.
3. Mash well after adding all the seasoning.
4. Put it in the fridge for ten minutes.
5. Now it is ready to be served with the food.

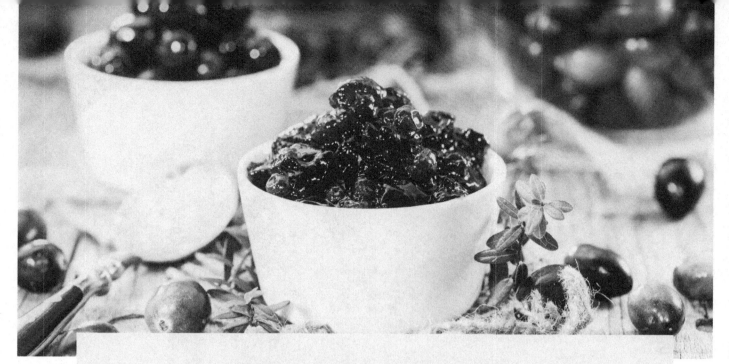

Cranberry Sauce

L&G count: 2 condiments

SERVINGS: 2   PREPPING TIME: 10 MINS   COOKING TIME: 20 MINS

Ingredients

One bag of cranberries

½ cup of water

One tsp of orange zest

Half tsp of vanilla

30 drops of sugar alternate

A pinch of salt

NUTRITION FACTS PER SERVES

Calories 110 kcal

Total Fat 0 gm

Total carbohydrates 6 gm

Protein 0 gm

Directions

1. Berries, zest, water, and seasoning should all be placed in a pan.
2. Cook on high heat till it boils, then turn the heat down and let it simmer until the berries explode.
3. Add vanilla and cook for a minute, then turn off the flame.
4. Let it sit for a while to cool.
5. When cool, serve with your favorite bread.

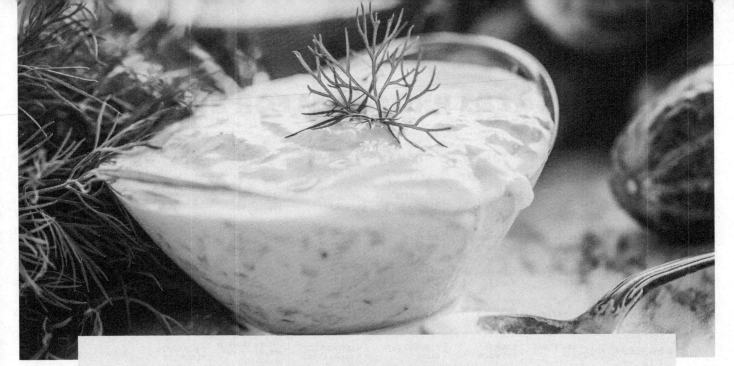

Killer Dip Recipe

L&G count: 2 condiments, 2 healthy fats

SERVINGS: 1   PREPPING TIME: 10 MINS   COOKING TIME: 0 MINS

Ingredients

Half cup of ricotta cheese

½ cup of Greek yogurt

One bsp of your favorite seasoning

NUTRITION FACTS PER SERVES

Calories 173 kcal

Total Fat 0 gm

Total carbohydrates 7 gm

Protein 16 gm

Directions

1. Using a spatula, mix the components inside a container and let the solution sit for an hour.
2. Enjoy it with any food, including vegetables.

PLAN 4&2&1 PROGRAM FOR 28 DAYS

WEEK 1	DAY 1	DAY 2	DAY 3	DAY 4	DAY 5	DAY 6	DAY 7
FUELING	HEAVEN CAULIFLOWER SALAD	LOBSTER TAIL	VEGETABLE BENEDICT	APPLE PEAR SHAKE	BAKED CINNAMON APPLES	FRENCH BARS	HEALTHY FRITTATA
FUELING	POMEGRANATE SALAD	CINNAMON PANCAKES	ZUCCHINI SPRING	NICOISE SALAD	TORTILLA AND TACO SALAD	FRESH ZUCCHINI NOODLES	CUCUMBER SALAD
FUELING	CHEDDAR BEEF BURGERS	BERRY YOGURT BAKE	BAKED CINNAMON APPLES	BANANA POPS	FRUIT QUINOA	QUICK EGGS AND HAM	STRAWBERRY YOGURT
FUELING	BERRY SHAKE	MIN MAC BEEF SALAD	STRAWBERRY YOGURT	BROCCOLI FRITTATA	FRESH ZUCCHINI NOODLES	CHIA PUDDING	FRUIT QUINOA
L&G MEAL	EGG AND TURKEY PIZZA	ROASTED RADISHES	POMEGRANATE SALAD	ROASTED BEET WHIT ORANGE	CHEESE STUFFED PEPPERS WITH BEEF	OVEN BAKED FLOUNDER	LOBSTER ROLL
L&G MEAL	ITALIAN CHICKEN	CREOLE CHICKEN	CHICKEN WHIT BROCCOLI	CHICKEN CHINESE CURRY	TUNA SALAD	BEEF STEW	BEEF WITH CROQUETTES
HEALTHY SNACKS	KALE CHIPS	RICED CAULIFLOWER	CARAMEL SCALLOPS	PROTEIN POT	PEPPERONI ROLL	CHEESE CAKE MUFFINS	FRENCH BARS

NOTES:

WEEK 2	DAY 1	DAY 2	DAY 3	DAY 4	DAY 5	DAY 6	DAY 7
FUELING	QUICK EGGS AND HAM	VEGETABLE BENEDICT	ISLAND SHAKE	APPLE PEAR SHAKE	BERRY SHAKE	FRUITY YOGURT	FRUIT QUINOA
FUELING	PUMPKIN PIE	RICED CAULIFLOWER	CARAMEL SCALLOPS	PROTEIN POT	AVOCADO DIP	KALE CHIPS	HONEY NUGGETS
FUELING	COCONUT PIE	BERRY PARFAIT	FRENCH BARS	PUMPKIN PIE	CHIA PUDDING	STRAWBERRY YOGURT	CHICKEN SOUP
FUELING	TUNA SALAD	TOFU BOWL	HEAVEN CAULIFLOWER SALAD	ROASTED RADISHES	SALMON DILL SALAD	NICOISE SALAD	EASY SHRIMP
L&G MEAL	BEEF STEW	CREOLE CHICKEN	MEXICAN MEATLOAF	FRESH ZUCCHINI NOODLES	CHICKEN SOUP	CRUSTY CAULIFLOWER PIE AND MEAT	LOBSTER ROLL
L&G MEAL	ITALIAN CHICKEN	SHRIMP WITH APPLE GREEN	LOBSTER TAIL	CHICKEN NOODLE ZUCCHINI	BAKED TILAPIA	BEEF STEW	CREAMY CHICKEN CASSEROLE
HEALTHY SNACKS	POMEGRANATE SALAD	KALE CHIPS	COCONUT PIE	CARAMEL SCALLOPS	PEPPERONI ROLL	BROCCOLI FRITTATA	FRENCH BARS

NOTES:

PLAN 4&2&1 PROGRAM FOR 28 DAYS

WEEK 3	DAY 1	DAY 2	DAY 3	DAY 4	DAY 5	DAY 6	DAY 7
FUELING	FRUIT QUINOA	CINNAMON PANCAKES (GLUTEN FREE)	BROCCOLI FRITTATA	QUICK EGGS AND HAM	TOAST WITH FRUITS AND EGG	CHEESY MUSHROOM OMELET	IRISH OATS AND NUTS
FUELING	PROTEIN POT	PUMPKIN PIE	CHIA PUDDING	STRAWBERRY YOGURT	HONEY OATS BAKED	TORTILLA AND TACO SALAD	FRESH ZUCCHINI NOODLES
FUELING	BERRY YOGURT BAKE	BAKED CINNAMON APPLES	BANANA POPS	ROASTED RADISHES	HEALTHY FRITTATA	EGGS WITH ASPARAGUS	MIN MAC BEEF SALAD
FUELING	COCONUT PIE	BROCCOLI FRITTATA	CUCUMBER SALAD	POMEGRANATE SALAD	ZUCCHINI SPRING	NICOISE SALAD	TORTILLA AND TACO SALAD
L&G MEAL	CHICKEN WITH BROCCOLI	ZUCCHINI SPRING	CHICKEN NOODLE ZUCCHINI	BAKED TILAPIA	VEGETABLE BURRITOS	CREOLE CHICKEN	CHEESE STUFFED PEPPERS WITH BEEF
L&G MEAL	BAKED TILAPIA	LOBSTER TAIL	CRUSTY CAULIFLOWER PIE	BAKED TILAPIA	SALMON SALAD	ITALIAN CHICKEN	CHEDDAR BEEF BURGERS
HEALTHY SNACKS	POMEGRANATE SALAD	PROTEIN POT	PEPPERONI ROLL	HONEY NUGGETS	FRENCH BARS	LEMON SANDWICH COOKIES	KALE CHIPS

NOTES:

WEEK 4	DAY 1	DAY 2	DAY 3	DAY 4	DAY 5	DAY 6	DAY 7
FUELING	QUICK EGGS AND HAM	FRUITY YOGURT	CINNAMON PANCAKES (GLUTEN FREE)	VEGETABLE BURRITOS	HEALTHY FRITTATA	CUCUMBER SALAD	BERRY YOGURT BAKE
FUELING	CHICKEN SOUP	FRUIT QUINOA	CHIA PUDDING	CHEER UP SHAKE	BERRY PARFAIT	COCONUT PIE	HONEY NUGGETS
FUELING	GINGERBREAD BISCUIT	LOW-CALORIE POPSICLE	FRENCH BARS	ROASTED BEET	NICOISE SALAD	STRAWBERRY YOGURT	CINNAMON PANCAKES (GLUTEN FREE)
FUELING	BERRY YOGURT BAKE	MIN MAC BEEF SALAD	FRESH ZUCCHINI NOODLES	FROZEN YOGURT BITES	STRAWBERRY CAKE	DARK CHOCOLATE MOUSE	CUCUMBER SALAD
L&G MEAL	LEMON TARRAGON COD	BAKED TILAPIA	CHICKEN SOUP	EGG AND TURKEY PIZZA	OVEN BAKED FLOUNDER	BAKED SNAPPER	PUMPKIN PIE
L&G MEAL	BAKED CHICKEN BREAST	BEEF STEW	SHRIMP WITH APPLE GREEN	BROILED LAMB CHOPS	CHEDDAR BEEF BURGERS	ORANGE BEEF WITH BROCCOLI	CHICKEN NOODLE ZUCCHINI
HEALTHY SNACKS	BANANA POPS	RICED CAULIFLOWER	PEPPERONI ROLL	FRENCH BARS	LOBSTER TAIL	HONEY OATS BAKED	KALE CHIPS

NOTES:

PLAN 5&1 PROGRAM FOR 28 DAYS

WEEK 1	DAY 1	DAY 2	DAY 3	DAY 4	DAY 5	DAY 6	DAY 7
FUELING	BROCCOLI FRITTATA	APPLE PEAR SHAKE	ROASTED RADISHES	FRUITY YOGURT	CUCUMBER SALAD	POMEGRANATE SALAD	QUICK EGGS AND HAM
FUELING	PROTEIN POT	STRAWBERRY CAKE	CHICKEN SOUP	FROZEN YOGURT BITES	HEALTHY FRITTATA	NICOISE SALAD	CHIA PUDDING
FUELING	BERRY SHAKE	MIN MAC BEEF SALAD	STRAWBERRY YOGURT	BROCCOLI FRITTATA	FRESH ZUCCHINI NOODLES	CHIA PUDDING	FRUIT QUINOA
FUELING	STRAWBERRY CAKE	LOBSTER TAIL	FRENCH BARS	EASY SHRIMP	CHEER UP SHAKE	MEXICAN MEATLOAF	BANANA POPS
FUELING	COCONUT PIE	BROCCOLI FRITTATA	CUCUMBER SALAD	POMEGRANATE SALAD	ZUCCHINI SPRING	NICOISE SALAD	TORTILLA AND TACO SALAD
L&G MEAL	ITALIAN CHICKEN	CHEDDAR BEEF BURGERS	VEGETABLE BURRITOS	CREOLE CHICKEN	QUICK EGGS AND HAM	OVEN BAKED FLOUNDER	CRUSTY CAULIFLOWER PIE

NOTES:

WEEK 2	DAY 1	DAY 2	DAY 3	DAY 4	DAY 5	DAY 6	DAY 7
FUELING	CUCUMBER SALAD	MEXICAN MEATLOAF	QUICK EGGS AND HAM	PUMPKIN PIE	BROCCOLI FRITTATA	CARAMEL SCALLOPS	COCONUT PIE
FUELING	EASY SHRIMP	PROTEIN POT	PEPPERONI ROLL	CHEER UP SHAKE	BERRY PARFAIT	BANANA POPS	HONEY OATS BAKED
FUELING	FRUIT QUINOA	CUCUMBER SALAD	ISLAND SHAKE	LEMON SANDWICH COOKIES	KALE CHIPS	EGGS WITH ASPARAGUS	PEPPERONI ROLL
FUELING	FRENCH BARS	HONEY NUGGETS	BERRY YOGURT BAKE	FRUITY YOGURT	ROASTED BEET WITH ORANGE	PUMPKIN PIE	ZUCCHINI SPRING
FUELING	TUNA SALAD	TOFU BOWL	HEAVEN CAULIFLOWER SALAD	ROASTED RADISHES	SALMON DILL SALAD	NICOISE SALAD	EASY SHRIMP
L&G MEAL	CHEDDAR BEEF BURGERS	HEALTHY FRITTATA	BEEF STEW	CRUSTY CAULIFLOWER PIE	BAKED TILAPIA	CHICKEN CHINESE CURRY	CHEESE STUFFED PEPPERS WITH BEEF

NOTES:

PLAN 5&1 PROGRAM FOR 28 DAYS

WEEK 3	DAY 1	DAY 2	DAY 3	DAY 4	DAY 5	DAY 6	DAY 7
FUELING	POMEGRANATE SALAD	RICED CAULIFLOWER	ROASTED RADISHES	SALMON DILL SALAD	ZUCCHINI SPRING	POMEGRANATE SALAD	QUICK EGGS AND HAM
FUELING	COCONUT PIE	BERRY PARFAIT	FRENCH BARS	PUMPKIN PIE	CHIA PUDDING	STRAWBERRY YOGURT	CHICKEN SOUP
FUELING	TUNA SALAD	TOFU BOWL	HEAVEN CAULIFLOWER SALAD	ROASTED RADISHES	SALMON DILL SALAD	NICOISE SALAD	EASY SHRIMP
FUELING	BANANA POPS	HEAVEN CAULIFLOWER SALAD	PEPPERONI ROLL	FRENCH BARS	LOBSTER TAIL	HONEY OATS BAKED	KALE CHIPS
FUELING	KALE CHIPS	RICED CAULIFLOWER	CARAMEL SCALLOPS	PROTEIN POT	PEPPERONI ROLL	CHEESE CAKE MUFFINS	FRENCH BARS
L&G MEAL	BEEF STEW	FRESH ZUCCHINI NOODLES	BAKED TILAPIA	CHICKEN CHINESE CURRY	CHICKEN SOUP	LOBSTER TAIL	ZUCCHINI SPRING

NOTES:

WEEK 4	DAY 1	DAY 2	DAY 3	DAY 4	DAY 5	DAY 6	DAY 7
FUELING	NICOISE SALAD	STRAWBERRY YOGURT	CHIA PUDDING	CHEER UP SHAKE	BERRY PARFAIT	COCONUT PIE	HONEY NUGGETS
FUELING	GINGERBREAD BISCUIT	LOW-CALORIE POPSICLE	FRENCH BARS	ROASTED BEET WITH ORANGE	NICOISE SALAD	STRAWBERRY YOGURT	CINNAMON PANCAKES
FUELING	TUNA SALAD	TOFU BOWL	HEAVEN CAULIFLOWER SALAD	ROASTED RADISHES	SALMON DILL SALAD	NICOISE SALAD	APPLE PEAR SHAKE
FUELING	KALE CHIPS	RICED CAULIFLOWER	CARAMEL SCALLOPS	PROTEIN POT	PEPPERONI ROLL	CHEESE CAKE MUFFINS	FRENCH BARS
FUELING	COCONUT PIE	BROCCOLI FRITTATA	CUCUMBER SALAD	POMEGRANATE SALAD	ZUCCHINI SPRING	FRUITY YOGURT	TORTILLA AND TACO SALAD
L&G MEAL	LEMON TARRAGON COD	LOBSTER TAIL	CRUSTY CAULIFLOWER PIE	BAKED TILAPIA	MEXICAN MEATLOAF	ITALIAN CHICKEN	CHEDDAR BEEF BURGERS

NOTES:

SPECIAL EXTRA CONTENT FOR YOU!

Conclusion

Feeling confident comes naturally when you maintain a balanced diet and a healthy body mass. It's the little things in life, like focusing on a healthy weight and diet, that can boost your confidence in your daily routine.

Imagine starting your day with a filling and nutritious breakfast; it sets the right tone for your morning and provides the energy you need. And when you start to feel a bit low, a healthy snack can refuel your body, keeping you going until your next meal.

Around two to three hours later, your body signals it's time for lunch, and having the right lean and green (L&G) foods assures productivity for the rest of the day. Following this routine builds confidence, allowing you to work with assurance throughout the day.

While many desire this confidence in their lives, they often struggle due to factors such as the cost and complexity of diet plans, believing they can't enjoy good food while dieting. However, this perspective changes with our diet plan. The novel encompasses a wide range of delectable cuisines, from sweets to shakes, chicken to vegetables, and healthy, delicious breakfast options. This plan challenges the notion that those on a diet cannot enjoy excellent food.

After reading this book, your perspective is likely different. Sharing this information is crucial; others can benefit and experience the same confidence in their lives that you've gained from a balanced diet and flavorful foods.

Your feedback on the website where you purchased the book would be greatly appreciated. Your guidance can help other readers make an informed decision and benefit from this sensible choice. Thank you for reading and considering our book.

INDEX

A

APPLE PEAR SHAKE...................................15
AVOCADO DIP..113

B

BAKED CHICKEN BREAST.........................62
BAKED CINNAMON APPLES......................82
BAKED SNAPPER 48
BAKED TILAPIA 49
BAKED VEGETABLE HUMMUS....................109
BANANA POPS..76
BEEF WITH CROQUETTES........................68
BEEF STEW..72
BEET FRUIT DIPPING...............................106
BEET SALAD WITH FETA.........................40
BERRY PARFAIT.......................................92
BERRY SHAKE..16
BERRY YOGURT BAKE.............................81
BLUEBERRY MINI CHEESE CAKE...............75
BROCCOLI FRITTATA................................24
BROILED LAMB CHOPS.............................71

C

CARAMEL SCALLOPS................................102
CHEDDAR BEEF BURGER..........................69
CHEER UP SHAKE....................................87
CHEESE CAKE MUFFINS...........................99
CHEESE STUFFED PEPPERS WITH BEEF.............70
CHEESY MUSHROOM OMELET....................23
CHIA PUDDING..85
CHICKEN CHINESE CURRY.......................63
CHICKEN NOODLE ZUCCHINI....................60
CHICKEN SOUP..56
CHICKEN WITH BROCCOLI.......................61

CHOCOLATE PUDDING WITH CHIA SEED......80
CINNAMON PANCAKES (GLUTEN FREE)...... 22
COCONUT PIE..93
CRAB SALAD IN AVOCADO.......................46
CRANBERRY SAUCE.................................114
CREAMY CHICKEN CASSEROLE.................58
CREOLE CHICKEN....................................59
CRUSTY CAULIFLOWER PIE AND MEAT.......66
CUCUMBER SALAD....................................27

D - E

DARK CHOCOLATE MOUSE.......................77
EASY SHRIMP..43
EGG AND TURKEY PIZZA.........................86
EGGS WITH ASPARAGUS.........................103

F-G

FRENCH BARS..89
FRESH ZUCCHINI NOODLES......................39
FROZEN YOGURT BITES...........................79
FRUIT QUINOA..19
FRUITY YOGURT.....................................18
GINGERBREAD BISCUIT............................91
GRILLED CHICKEN MARINATED WITH BEER..57

H-I- K

HEALTHY FRITTATA.................................11
HEALTHY QUICK CUCUMBER SALAD..........41
HEAVEN CAULIFLOWER SALAD.................38
HONEY MUSTARD SAUCE.........................111
HONEY NUGGETS....................................97
HONEY OATS BAKED...............................95
IRISH OATS AND NUTS...........................20

ISLAND SHAKE................................14

ITALIAN CHICKEN............................55

KALE CHIPS...............................101

KILLER DIP RECIPE........................115

L - M

LEMON SANDWICH COOKIES......................96

LEMON TARRAGON COD..........................44

LOBSTER ROLL...............................50

LOBSTER TAIL...............................45

LOW-CALORIE POPSICLE 94

MEXICAN MEATLOAF...........................65

MIN MAC BEEF SALAD........................ 73

N - O

NICOISE SALAD..............................29

OMELETTE WITH PEPPERS AND MUSHROOMS........17

ORANGE BEEF WITH BROCCOLI..................67

OVEN BAKED FLOUNDER 47

P - Q

PEANUT BUTTER ENERGY BALLS.................88

PEPPERONI ROLL 108

POMEGRANATE SALAD..........................36

PROTEIN POT...............................105

PUMPKIN PIE................................90

PURPLE KOHLRABI WITH ORANGE................34

QUICK EGGS AND HAM.........................12

R

RED PEPPER AND CHICK PEA DIP..............104

RED PEPPER SAUCE..........................112

RICED CAULIFLOWER........................107

ROASTED ASPARAGUS WITH GARLIC............35

ROASTED BEET WITH ORANGE.................33

ROASTED RADISHES.........................37

S

SALMON DILL SALAD.........................30

SALMON SALAD.............................53

SHRIMP WITH APPLE GREEN..................52

STRAWBERRY CAKE..........................83

STRAWBERRY YOGURT........................78

T

TOAST WITH FRUITS AND EGG................21

TOFU BOWL...............................31

TORTILLA AND TACO SALAD.................28

TUNA SALAD..............................51

V- Y

VEGETABLE BENEDICT......................13

VEGETABLE BURRITOS......................25

YOGURT AND PUMPKIN DIP.................. 100

Z

ZUCCHINI SPRING.........................32

Made in the USA
Columbia, SC
18 December 2024